MW00625366

EMRA
Ortho Guide

Editors-in-Chief
Sepehr Sedigh Haghighat, MD
Robert Hsu, MD, FACEP
Jeremy Berberian, MD

Associate Editors
W. Brandon White, DO
Mahesh Polavarapu, MD

2018–2019 EMRA Board of Directors

Omar Maniya, MD, MBA | President
Hannah Hughes, MD, MBA | President-Elect
Zach Jarou, MD | Immediate Past President
Tommy Eales, DO | Secretary/Editor, EM Resident
Nathan Vafaie, MD, MBA | Speaker of the Council
Karina Sanchez, MD | Vice-Speaker of the Council
Erik Blutinger, MD, MSc | Resident Representative to ACEP
Sara Paradise Dimeo, MD | Director of Education
Angela Cai, MD, MBA | Director of Health Policy
Greg Tanquary, DO, MBA | Director of Membership
Nick Salerno, MD | Director of Technology
Eric McDonald, MD | ACGME RC-EM Liaison
Breanne Jaqua, DO | ACGME RC-EM Liaison
Venkat Subramanyam, MD | Ex-Officio Board Member
Scott Pasichow, MD, MPH | EMRA Representative to AMA
Corey McNeilly, MA | Medical Student Council Chair

EMRA Reviewers

Sara Paradise Dimeo, MD
Richard Grantier III, MD
Venkat Subramanyam, MD
Jonathon Pickos, DO

EMRA Staff

Cathey B. Wise, CAE | Executive Director
Valerie Hunt | Managing Editor

Peer Reviewers

Brian J. Levine, MD, FACEP
Daniel M. Grawl, PA-C

Images

Medical Illustrations by Body Render
Radiographs courtesy of Christiana
Care Health System

DISCLAIMER

Foreword

Traumatic injuries are a common presentation in emergency departments, urgent care centers, and outpatient settings. Yet, because of the lack of required training during medical school, the care and management of acute musculoskeletal injuries is often foreign to new trainees and providers in acute care settings. Furthermore, many currently available references are geared toward orthopedic providers and focused on surgical management. Our ED has the benefit of being a high-volume Level I trauma and tertiary referral center without an orthopedic surgery residency. As a result, our EM teams manage thousands of fracture injuries annually, and this book is the brainchild of several residents and faculty who were looking for information geared toward helping acute care providers manage these common injuries.

Our goal is to provide you with an easy reference to help you care for patients with acute orthopedic injuries. As with most clinical medicine, treatment and practice patterns will vary with institutional culture. However, this guide aims to offer you a foundation to build upon as you see more and more traumatic bony injuries. This text is not intended to provide comprehensive management guidelines for every injury; each of the chapters in this book include bones and joints that are treated by specialized surgeons who have spent years in residency and fellowship training.

We have included fracture basics as an introduction on "how to speak orthopedics," and we've outlined key splinting techniques and neurologic examination findings. Importantly, we have also provided common fracture/joint reduction techniques and tips for reference to help you in your practice.

Lastly, we would like to thank all the residents and faculty at Christiana Care, orthopedic colleagues, and editorial staff who helped create this unique resource. Many of us graduated from medical school with minimal knowledge or experience in assessing and managing orthopedic injuries. We hope this guide will help those in similar shoes!

Sincerely,
Editors of the EMRA Ortho Guide
Department of Emergency Medicine
Emergency Medicine Residency
Christiana Care Health System

Contributors

Fracture Basics
Sepehr Sedigh Haghighat, MD
Robert Hsu, MD, FACEP
Mahesh Polavarapu, MD
Christiana Care Health System

Cervical Spine
Melissa V. Cummings, MD
Christiana Care Health System

Thoracolumbar Spine
Gillian Bach, MD
University of Pennsylvania

Thorax
Lauren Briskie, MD
Christiana Care Health System

Shoulder and Arm
Sepehr Sedigh Haghighat, MD
Christiana Care Health System

Elbow
Jonathan A. Hilton, MD
Christiana Care Health System

Forearm and Wrist
W. Brandon White, DO
Sepehr Sedigh Haghighat, MD
Christiana Care Health System

Hand
Genna A. Jerrard, MD
Christiana Care Health System

Pelvis and Femur
Daniel Kreider, MD
Adam Quinn, MD
Christiana Care Health System

Knee and Leg
Michael Murphey, MD
Ryan D. Gordon, MD
Christiana Care Health System

Ankle
Sushant Kapoor, DO, MS
Christiana Care Health System

Foot
Mahesh Polavarapu, MD
Kyle Burch, MD
Christiana Care Health System

Splinting
Robert Hsu, MD, FACEP
Christiana Care Health System

Neurologic Exam
Mahesh Polavarapu, MD
W. Brandon White, DO
Christiana Care Health System

Table of Contents

Chapter 5. Shoulder and Arm

Chapter 6. Elbow

Chapter 7. Forearm and Wrist

Chapter 10. Knee and Leg

Chapter 11. Ankle

Chapter 14. Neurologic Exam

CHAPTER 1

Fracture Basics

HOW TO DESCRIBE A FRACTURE

- Open vs. Closed
  - Based on clinical exam, sometimes in conjunction with imaging
  - See Open Fractures section
- Fracture Types
  - Complete: all the way through the bone
    - **Transverse**: runs perpendicular to the long axis of the bone
    - **Oblique**: runs diagonally to the long axis of the bone
    - **Spiral**: corkscrew-shaped fracture resulting from rotational/torsional force
    - **Comminuted**: > 2 fracture fragments
  - Incomplete (Ⓟ Peds): the entire cortex is not broken
    - **Bowing**: bending of a long bone without returning to its original position
    - **Torus/Buckle**: bulging of the cortex, typically at the metaphysis, resulting from axial compression

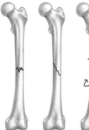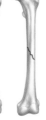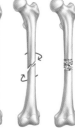

Transverse   Oblique   Spiral   Comminuted

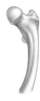

Greenstick   Buckle   Bow

- **Greenstick**: fracture of the cortex on just one side of the bone
- — Salter-Harris: fractures that involve the growth plate (see p. 5)
- Fracture Location
  - — **Long bones**: proximal, middle, distal
  - — ⓟ Pediatric
    - **Diaphysis**: shaft
    - **Metaphysis**: widened parts at ends of bones adjacent to physis
    - **Physis**: radiolucent growth plate between metaphysis and epiphysis

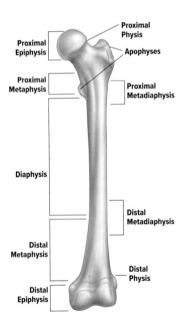

Proximal Physis

Proximal Epiphysis

Apophyses

Proximal Metaphysis

Proximal Metadiaphysis

Diaphysis

Distal Metadiaphysis

Distal Metaphysis

Distal Physis

Distal Epiphysis

- **Epiphysis**: secondary ossification center at the end of bones
- **Apophysis**: secondary ossification center at site of tendon or ligament attachment
— Anatomical name (such as base, shaft, neck, or head of the metacarpals)
- Displacement
  — **Note**: Displacement is a broad term that describes the movement of fracture fragments (distal relative to proximal) and includes all of the following terms but is commonly used to describe just translation.
  — **Angulation/alignment**: describes extent of angulation relative to the long axis of the bone
    - **Valgus**: lateral angulation
    - **Varus**: medial angulation
  — **Apposition**: describes the amount of contact between the ends of the fracture fragments
    - **Bayonet apposition**: used to describe when fracture fragments are aligned side by side
  — **Distraction**: describes when fragments are pulled apart
  — **Impaction**: describes when fragments are pushed together
  — **Translation**: describes extent of movement perpendicular to long axis of the bone, typically as a percentage the bone's width
  — **Rotation**: describes extent of rotation of the distal fracture fragment relative to the proximal portion (often clinically apparent)
- **Concurrent injuries**: include joint involvement and/or additional fractures
  — Evaluate at least one joint above and below, clinically +/- imaging

OPEN FRACTURES

Definition
- Fracture with direct communication to external environment
- Classified as Gustilo I, II, III

General Management in the ED
- Hemostasis
  — Direct pressure to control bleeding (be aware of sharp bone)
  — If tourniquet is required:
    - Place tourniquet above the wound, as distal as possible, while avoiding joints
    - Tighten the tourniquet only until bleeding stops
    - Document before/after tourniquet exam and time tourniquet was placed
- Assessment
  — Thorough physical exam that includes assessment for soft tissue damage, vascular injuries, and neurologic injuries (see Chapter 14)
- Debridement and irrigation with saline
- Dressing
  — Remove gross debris from wound
  — Place sterile saline-soaked dressing over the wound
- Stabilize
  — Splint fracture for temporary stabilization to decrease pain and prevent further injury
- Antibiotics
  — Tetanus prophylaxis and IV antibiotics (consider 1st generation cephalosporin +/- aminoglycoside or piperacillin/tazobactam for farm injuries or possible bowel contamination)

SALTER-HARRIS CLASSIFICATION (Ⓟ PEDS)

- Most widely used classification system to describe physeal fractures in children
- Management includes adequate reduction of the fracture, splinting, non-weight bearing, orthopedic consultation
  — Type III-V often require surgical management

Type I	• Transverse fracture through the growth plate (physis) • Tenderness over physis should be a presumed SH I • May be missed on initial plain films
Type II	• Fracture through physis and metaphysis • Most common Salter-Harris fracture
Type III	• Fracture through physis and epiphysis involving the articular surface
Type IV	• Fracture through metaphysis, physis, and epiphysis involving the articular surface
Type V	• Compression fracture of the growth plate (physis) • Often missed or thought to be Salter-Harris I • Suspect if mechanism of injury involves a significant axial load • Often diagnosed retrospectively after arrest of growth has developed

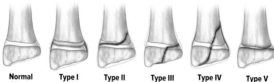

Normal   Type I   Type II   Type III   Type IV   Type V
Physis

NON-ACCIDENTAL TRAUMA (NAT)

- General findings concerning for NAT
  - Long bone fractures in non-ambulatory child
  - Multiple fractures, especially if in various stages of healing
  - Metaphyseal fractures
    - Corner fractures
    - Bucket handle fractures
  - Avulsion fractures
  - Transverse fractures
- Specific fractures concerning for NAT
  - Femur fractures
  - Rib fractures, especially posterior
  - Scapular fractures
  - Skull fractures
  - Vertebral body and/or spinous process fractures
- Considerations in NAT
  - Diaphyseal callus forms 5–14 days after fracture
  - Distal tibial spiral/oblique fractures in ambulatory children are typically not NAT

CHAPTER 2

Cervical Spine

FRACTURES BY LOCATION

Posterior View

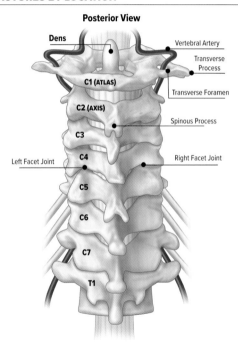

Dens

Vertebral Artery

Transverse Process

C1 (ATLAS)

Transverse Foramen

C2 (AXIS)

Spinous Process

C3

Left Facet Joint — C4 — Right Facet Joint

C5

C6

C7

T1

EVALUATION

- In a patient with concerning mechanism for C-spine injury, assume injury and apply a cervical collar if unable to immediately evaluate for C-spine injury
- C-spine clearance can be accomplished radiographically or by clinical evaluation (eg, NEXUS criteria or Canadian C-Spine Rules)
  - Delayed clearance can lead to increased risk of pressure sores, increased work of breathing, aspiration, and pain
  - High-risk populations include patients with rheumatoid arthritis, Down syndrome, cervical hardware
- Radiographic evaluation must include bottom of T1 vertebra
- Unstable C-spine fractures ("Jefferson Bit Off A Hangman's Thumb")
  - **J**efferson fracture
  - **B**ilateral facet dislocations
  - **O**dontoid fractures, Types II and III
  - **A**tlanto-occipital dissociation
  - **H**angman's fracture
  - **T**eardrop fracture, flexion type

C-spine Radiographic Considerations

X-Ray	CT	MRI	CTA/MRA
Indicated only if CT unavailable	Ideal modality for detecting fractures and dislocations	Indicated for neurologic and ligamentous evaluation	Indicated for vascular evaluation
Less radiation	More radiation	No radiation	Variable radiation
Moderate sensitivity for significant injuries	No significant fractures missed	Best to visualize soft tissue, ligaments, intervertebral discs, spinal cord, spinal epidural hematomas	Best to evaluate for vertebral artery injury

℗ Pediatric Considerations

- Three-view X-ray has high sensitivity to rule out C-spine fractures
- In children < 8 years old, ligamentous injuries are more common than fractures
- Clinical decision rules
  — NEXUS criteria have been validated to patients as young as 8 years old
  — Canadian C-spine rules did not include pediatric patients in their study

ATLANTO-OCCIPITAL DISSOCIATION (AOD)

General

- Disruption of all ligamentous connections between occiput and C1 (atlas)
  — Includes dislocation and subluxation
  — Highly unstable and often fatal
- Mechanism: severe hyperextension injury with distraction
  — Non-traumatic AOD may occur in patients with Down syndrome and rheumatoid arthritis
- Classified by complete vs. incomplete ligamentous disruption

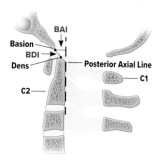

Associated Injuries

- Lower cranial nerve (VI, X, XII) dysfunction
- Lower brain stem injury leading to respiratory arrest
- Disruption of tectorial ligaments

Radiographic Evaluation

- AP, lateral, and odontoid views
  — Basion-dens interval (BDI) or basion-axial interval (BAI) > 12 mm suggests injury
- CT (ideal modality)

- Consider CTA and MRI to evaluate for vascular and ligamentous/neurologic injuries

Management
- Immobilization in cervical collar
  - Especially important to avoid flexion and axial traction

Disposition
- Discuss with spine specialist while patient is in the ED
  - Almost always requires surgical management

BILATERAL CERVICAL FACET DISLOCATION

General
- Disruption of the cervical facets that connect the adjacent vertebrae leading to instability and possible vertebral dislocation
  - Commonly occur between C5–C7
- Mechanism: hyperflexion and/or flexion-distraction
- Exam: inability to move head

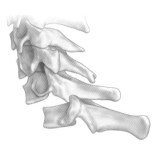

Associated Injuries
- Neurologic injury common
  - Spinal cord injury (see Chapter 14)
  - C6 and/or C7 radiculopathy (see Chapter 14)

Radiographic Evaluation
- AP and lateral views
- CT (ideal modality)
- Consider MRI to evaluate for ligamentous/neurologic injuries

Management
- Immobilization in cervical collar

Disposition
- Discuss with spine specialist while patient is in the ED
  - Almost always requires surgical management

C1 ARCH (ATLAS) FRACTURE

General
- Fracture of the anterior or posterior arch of C1
- Mechanism: typically hyperextension

Associated Injuries
- Anterior arch fractures: soft tissue swelling
- Posterior arch fractures: other C-spine fractures, especially the dens

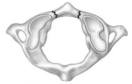

Anterior Arch Fracture

Radiographic Evaluation
- AP, lateral, and odontoid views
  - For Ⓟ pediatric patients, assess atlanto-dens interval (ADI) on lateral view (normal is < 5 mm)
- CT (ideal modality)
- Consider MRI to evaluate for ligamentous/neurologic injuries

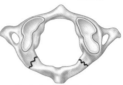

Posterior Arch Fracture

Management
- Immobilization in cervical collar

Disposition
- Discuss with spine specialist while patient is in the ED
  - Almost always requires surgical management

CERVICAL BURST FRACTURE

General
- Subaxial (below C1) cervical vertebral body fracture that extends through the posterior cortex
  — May have fracture fragments that are displaced into the spinal canal
- Mechanism: high energy axial loading

Associated Injuries
- Spinal cord injury (see Chapter 14)
- Posterior ligament injury
  — If ligament injury present, can cause cord compression with complete or incomplete spinal cord injury

Radiographic Evaluation
- AP, lateral, and odontoid views
- CT (ideal modality)
- Consider MRI to evaluate for ligamentous/neurologic injuries

Management
- Immobilization in cervical collar

Disposition
- Discuss with spine specialist while patient is in the ED
  — Often requires surgical management

EXTENSION TEARDROP FRACTURE

General
- Avulsion fracture of the anteroinferior aspect of the vertebral body without associated loss of vertebral height as commonly seen with flexion teardrop injuries
  — Commonly occurs at C2
- Mechanism: forced hyperextension

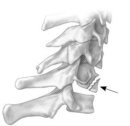

Associated Injuries
- Central cord syndrome (see Chapter 14)

Radiographic Evaluation

- AP and lateral views
- CT (ideal modality)
- Consider MRI to evaluate for ligamentous/neurologic injuries

Management

- Immobilization in cervical collar

Disposition

- Discuss with spine specialist while patient is in the ED
  — Almost always requires surgical management

FLEXION TEARDROP FRACTURE

General

- Complete ligamentous disruption along with comminuted vertebral body fracture and facet joint disruption
  — Typically occurs at C5–C6
- Mechanism: axial compression and hyperflexion (eg, headfirst dive into shallow water)

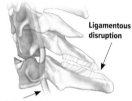

Ligamentous disruption

Spinal Cord

Associated Injuries

- Quadriplegia
- Anterior cord syndrome (see Chapter 14)

Radiographic Evaluation

- AP and lateral views
- CT (ideal modality)
- Consider CTA and MRI to evaluate for vascular and neurologic/ligamentous injuries

Management

- Immobilization in cervical collar

Disposition

- Discuss with spine specialist while patient is in the ED
  — Almost always requires surgical management

HANGMAN'S FRACTURE

General
- Traumatic spondylolisthesis of C2 (axis) with fracture of C2 pedicles and anterior displacement of C2 on C3
- Mechanism: hyperextension with vertical compression injury
  - Classically associated with hangings, now typically seen in MVCs
  - **℗ Pediatrics:** combination of flexion and distraction (rare in children < 8 years old)
- Classified as Levine and Edwards Type I–III

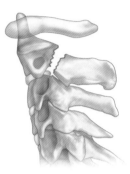

Type II Hangman's Fracture

Associated Injuries
- Concurrent C-spine fractures
- Low incidence of cord injury

Radiographic Evaluation
- AP, lateral, and odontoid views
- CT (ideal modality)
- Consider CTA and MRI to evaluate for vascular and neurologic/ligamentous injuries

Management
- Immobilization in cervical collar

Disposition
- Discuss with spine specialist while patient is in the ED
  - Almost always requires surgical management

JEFFERSON FRACTURE

General

- Burst fracture of C1 (atlas)
  - Fractures of left and right anterior and posterior arches
  - Stability based on ligament stability (specifically transverse and alar ligaments)
- Unstable if:
  - Displacement of C1 lateral masses > 7 mm
  - Avulsion includes entire anterior arch
- Mechanism: axial load and/or hyperextension
- In Ⓟ pediatric patients, fracture proceeds through open synchondroses, and may occur with minimal trauma
  - Posterior synchondrosis fuses at age 4
  - Anterior synchondrosis fuses at age 7

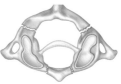
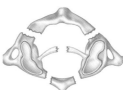

Axial View

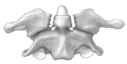

Coronal View

Associated Injuries

- Other cervical spine fractures
- Vertebral artery injuries
  - Can lead to lateral medullary (Wallenberg) syndrome
- Ligamentous injuries

Radiographic Evaluation

- AP, lateral, and odontoid views
  - Odontoid view demonstrates overlapping C1 and C2 facets
- CT (ideal modality)
- Consider CTA and MRI to evaluate for vascular and neurologic/ligamentous injuries

Management

- Immobilization in cervical collar

Disposition
- Discuss with spine specialist while patient is in the ED
  — Almost always requires surgical management

ODONTOID (DENS/PEG) FRACTURE

General
- Fracture of the dens (peg) of the axis (C2)
  — Most common upper cervical spine fracture
- Mechanism
  — Hyperflexion (majority of injuries) leads to anterior displacement of dens
  — Hyperextension leads to posterior displacement of dens
- Classified as Type I, II, or III
  — **Type I**: fracture of the upper part of the odontoid, rare, considered stable
  — **Type II**: fracture at the base of the odontoid, most common, unstable
  — **Type III**: fracture through the odontoid and into the lateral masses of C2, unstable

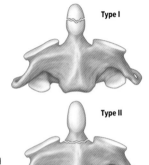

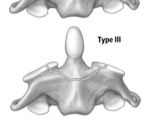

Associated Injuries
- Types II and III associated with atlas injury
- Type II associated with vascular injury
- Transverse ligament failure leading to atlantoaxial instability
- C2-C3 pseudosubluxation can be seen in young children

Radiographic Evaluation

- AP, lateral and open mouth views
  - For pediatric patients, evaluate Swischuk line on lateral view: runs anteriorly from posterior arch of C1 to posterior arch of C3
  - Subluxation likely if posterior arch of C2 ≥ 2 mm from this line
- CT (ideal modality)
- Consider CTA and MRI to evaluate for vascular and neurologic/ligamentous injuries

Management

- Immobilization in cervical collar

Disposition

- Discuss with spine specialist while patient is in the ED
  - Types II and III almost always require surgical management

EMRA Ortho Guide

CHAPTER 3

Thoracolumbar Spine

FRACTURES BY LOCATION

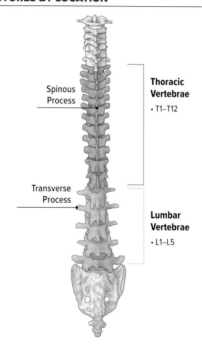

Spinous Process

Transverse Process

Thoracic Vertebrae
• T1–T12

Lumbar Vertebrae
• L1–L5

ANATOMICAL 3-COLUMN CONCEPT OF THE SPINE

- Spine divided into 3 columns: anterior, middle, and posterior
- Stability requires at least 2 of 3 columns intact

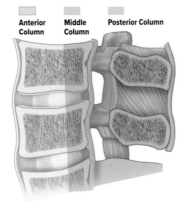

Anterior Column — **Middle Column** — **Posterior Column**

Anterior Column	Middle Column	Posterior Column
• Anterior Longitudinal Ligament (ALL) • Anterior 2/3 of the vertebral body and intervertebral disc (annulus fibrosus)	• Posterior Longitudinal Ligament (PLL) • Posterior 1/3 of the vertebral body and intervertebral disc (annulus fibrosus)	• Ligamentum flavum • Posterior Ligament Complex • Pedicles • Lamina • Facets • Spinous process

BURST FRACTURE

General
- Unstable comminuted fracture of the vertebral body
  - Posterior body fractures can lead to retropulsion of bony fragments into spinal canal
- Mechanism: axial compression

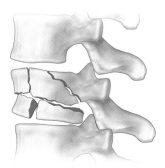

Associated Injuries
- Posterior ligament injury
- Spinal cord injury, especially if posterior column involved (see Chapter 14)

Radiographic Evaluation
- AP and lateral views
- CT (ideal modality)
- Consider MRI to evaluate for neurologic/ligamentous injuries

Management
- Immobilization in TLSO (Thoracic Lumbar Sacral Orthosis) for stable fractures without neurologic injury

Disposition
- Discuss with spine specialist while patient is in the ED
  - Often requires surgical management

CHANCE FRACTURE (FLEXION-DISTRACTION)

General

- Unstable horizontal fracture through the vertebra, most commonly in the upper lumbar spine, typically involving all 3 columns
  - Chance fracture without ligamentous injury is known as a "bony Chance fracture"
- Mechanism: hyperflexion and distraction of the spine

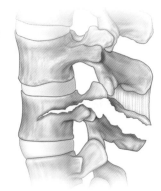

Associated Injuries

- Neurologic deficits if posterior column involved (see Chapter 14)
- High incidence of gastrointestinal injury

Radiographic Evaluation

- AP and lateral views
- CT (ideal modality)
- Consider MRI to evaluate for neurologic/ligamentous injuries

Management

- Spinal immobilization

Disposition

- Discuss with spine specialist while patient is in the ED
  - Almost always requires surgical management

FRACTURE DISLOCATION

General
- Unstable injury involving all 3 columns and ligamentous disruption
- Most commonly occurs at the thoracolumbar junction (T10–L2)
- Mechanism: shearing force

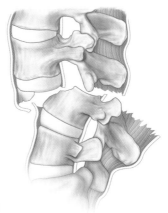

Associated Injuries
- High incidence of spinal cord injuries (see Chapter 14)

Radiographic Evaluation
- AP and lateral views
- CT (ideal modality)
- Consider MRI to evaluate for ligamentous and/or spinal cord injury

Management
- Spinal immobilization

Disposition
- Discuss with spine specialist while patient is in the ED
  — Almost always requires surgical management

TRANSVERSE PROCESS, SPINOUS PROCESS, AND PARS INTERARTICULARIS FRACTURES

General
- Fractures of the transverse process, spinous process, and/or pars interarticularis
- Mechanism: direct trauma

Associated Injuries
- One type of fracture increases the risk of others in this group
- Neurologic injury is uncommon

Radiographic Evaluation

- AP, lateral, and lateral oblique views
- CT (ideal modality)

Management

- Conservative management

Disposition

- ED discharge and follow-up with orthopedic specialist

WEDGE COMPRESSION FRACTURE

General

- Compression fracture involving collapse of the anterior vertebral body
  - Considered unstable if involvement of posterior structures, multiple adjacent wedge fractures, or loss of anterior vertebral height > 50%
- Mechanism: flexion with axial compression

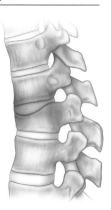

Associated Injuries

- Neurologic deficits (see Chapter 14)
- Impaired pulmonary function with thoracic injuries

Radiographic Evaluation

- AP and lateral views
- CT spine (ideal modality)

Management

- Conservative management

Disposition

- Discuss with spine specialist while patient is in the ED for unstable fractures, neurologic injury, or impaired pulmonary function
  - Often requires surgical management
- ED discharge and follow-up with spine specialist for uncomplicated stable fractures

CHAPTER 4

Thorax

FRACTURES BY LOCATION

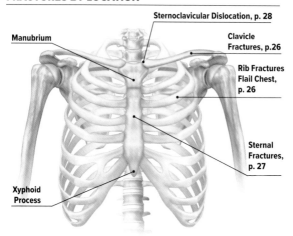

Sternoclavicular Dislocation, p. 28

Clavicle Fractures, p.26

Rib Fractures Flail Chest, p. 26

Manubrium

Sternal Fractures, p. 27

Xyphoid Process

CLAVICULAR FRACTURE

General
- Three types
  - Type I: middle 1/3 of clavicle (75–80% of clavicular fractures)
  - Type II: lateral 1/3 of clavicle (10–15% of clavicular fractures)
  - Type III: medial 1/3 of clavicle

Associated Injuries
- Middle 1/3 fractures
  - Subclavian artery/vein injury
  - Contusion or avulsion of nerve roots, brachial plexus injury (see Chapter 14)
- Lateral 1/3 fractures
  - Coracoclavicular ligament damage
  - AC joint dislocation or subluxation
- Medial 1/3 fractures
  - Intrathoracic injuries
  - Rib and sternal fractures

Radiographic Evaluation
- Clavicle AP and AP views with cephalic angulation
  - Consider serendipity view (45° cephalic angulation) to better visualize the sternoclavicular joint
- Consider CT for complicated fractures

Management
- Immobilization in sling or shoulder immobilizer
- Indications for surgical management: open fracture, displaced fracture with skin tenting, neurovascular injuries, floating shoulder (distal clavicle and scapula neck fracture with > 10 mm displacement), shortening > 2 cm in pediatric patient

Disposition
- ED discharge and follow-up with orthopedic specialist if no indications for surgical management

RIB FRACTURES/FLAIL CHEST

General
- Most common bony injury in chest trauma
- Flail chest: 3 or more adjacent ribs with segmental fractures
  - Exam characterized by paradoxical chest wall motion

Associated Injuries
- Pneumothorax, hemothorax, pulmonary contusion
- Intra-abdominal injury
- Vascular injury
- 1st and 2nd rib fractures associated with blunt cardiac injury, bronchial tears, major vascular injuries

Radiographic Evaluation
- AP and lateral views or rib series (low sensitivity)
- CT (ideal modality)

Management
- Respiratory support, incentive spirometry, multimodal pain control

Disposition
- Discuss with trauma specialist while patient is in the ED
  - Flail chest and geriatric patients with multiple rib fractures almost always require admission

STERNAL FRACTURE

General
- Sternal body fracture most common
- Mechanism: High-energy trauma

Associated Injuries
- Blunt cardiac injury (BCI)
  - Low incidence of clinically significant cardiac dysrhythmias

Radiographic Evaluation
- CT (ideal modality)

Management
- Initial EKG and cardiac biomarkers with repeat in 6 hours
  - No further workup for BCI if normal initial vital signs, no abnormalities on initial and repeat EKG, and normal initial and repeat cardiac biomarkers

Disposition
- ED discharge and follow-up with orthopedic specialist if isolated fracture with no evidence of BCI

STERNOCLAVICULAR DISLOCATION

General

- Traumatic dislocation, most common anteriorly, with high incidence of concurrent significant injuries
  — Atraumatic subluxation can be seen in younger patients

Associated Injuries

- Anterior dislocations: pneumothorax, hemothorax, pulmonary contusion, rib fractures
- Posterior dislocations: tracheal injury, pneumothorax, subclavian vein compression, SVC laceration (orthopedic emergency)

Radiographic Evaluation

- Sternoclavicular PA and anterior oblique views
  — Consider serendipity view (45° cephalic angulation) to better visualize the sternoclavicular joint
- CT (ideal modality)

Management

- Anterior dislocation: reduction followed by pressure bandage to maintain stability
- Posterior dislocation: if patient stable, do NOT attempt immediate reduction as clavicle may be tamponading vascular injury

Sternoclavicular Reduction Technique

Steps	First Person	Second Person
1	Place folded sheet between shoulders with patient supine	AB-duct the arm and apply traction
2	Anterior dislocation: Downward force on clavicle Posterior dislocation: Pull clavicle anteriorly	

Disposition

- Discuss with orthopedic specialist while patient is in the ED
  — Often requires surgical management

Shoulder and Arm

FRACTURES BY LOCATION

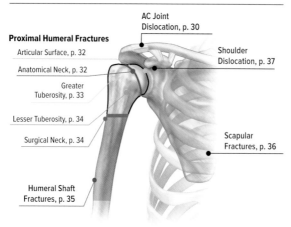

ACROMIOCLAVICULAR (AC) JOINT DISLOCATION

General
- Dissociation, subluxation, or dislocation of the clavicle from the scapula
  - The two bones are held together by AC and CC (coracoclavicular) ligaments
- Mechanism: usually direct force from above or FOOSH
- Exam: pain worse with AC-cross-arm AD-duction test (bringing the arm across the body and almost trying to touch the opposite shoulder with forearm)
- Classified as Types I-VI by severity of ligamentous injury

Associated Injuries
- Shoulder dislocation

Radiographic Evaluation
- AP views
  - AC joint width should be < 3-5 mm
  - CC distance (from clavicle to superior coracoid process) should be < 13 mm in adults
  - Clavicle should be level with the acromion

Management
- Immobilization in sling

Disposition
- ED discharge and follow-up with orthopedic specialist
  - Severe injuries may require surgical management

PROXIMAL HUMERUS FRACTURE

General

- Fracture involving the humeral head from articular surface to surgical neck (below the lesser and greater tuberosity)
  - Usually involves older population

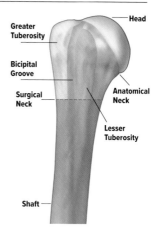

- Mechanism: FOOSH or direct trauma
- Exam: pain that is worse with movement, typically external rotation
- Further subcategorization
  - Anatomic neck fractures
  - Articular surface fractures
  - Combination fractures
  - Greater tuberosity fractures
  - Lesser tuberosity fractures
  - Surgical neck fractures
- Classified as Neer 1-4
  - Determined by number of fracture fragments and level of displacement (angulation > 45° or displacement > 1 cm)
  - Does not include articular surface fractures
  - Guides treatment and prognosis

Anatomic Neck Fracture (Proximal Humerus Fracture)

General
- Bimodal distribution: adults and adolescents (typically 8–14 years old)

Associated Injuries
- High incidence of avascular necrosis

Radiographic Evaluation
- AP and lateral views

Management
- Immobilization in sling

Disposition
- Discuss with orthopedic specialist while patient is in the ED
  - Displaced fractures will often require surgical management

Articular Surface Fracture (Proximal Humerus Fracture)

General
- Also called impression fractures

Associated Injuries
- Anterior and posterior shoulder dislocations
- Avascular necrosis with comminuted fractures

Radiographic Evaluation
- AP views in internal and external rotation
  - Fat fluid level on AP upright view suggests articular surface fracture

Management
- Immobilization in sling with arm in external rotation

Disposition
- Discuss with orthopedic specialist while patient is in the ED

Combination Fracture (Proximal Humerus Fracture)

General
- Severely comminuted and displaced 3-part or 4-part fractures

Associated Injuries
- Shoulder dislocations
- Rotator cuff injuries
- Brachial plexus, axillary vessels, axillary and musculocutaneous nerve injuries (see Chapter 14)
- Avascular necrosis of the humeral head

Radiographic Evaluation
- AP, lateral, and scapular Y views

Management
- Immobilization in sling

Disposition
- Discuss with orthopedic specialist while patient is in the ED
  — Almost always requires surgical management

Greater Tuberosity Fracture (Proximal Humerus Fracture)

General
- Displacement defined as ≥ 0.5 cm

Associated Injuries
- Displaced fractures: rotator cuff injuries and anterior shoulder dislocations

Radiographic Evaluation
- AP view to assess for superior displacement and axillary view to assess for posterior displacement
- Consider CT to better evaluate displacement

Management
- Immobilization in sling
- If anterior dislocation present, reduction will often correct displacement, after which it can be treated as a non-displaced fracture

Disposition
- Displaced fracture: Discuss with orthopedic specialist while patient is in the ED
- Non-displaced fracture: ED discharge and follow-up with orthopedic specialist

Lesser Tuberosity Fracture (Proximal Humerus Fracture)

General
- Isolated fractures uncommon and often missed
- Mechanism: fall on AB-ducted arm or seizure

Associated Injuries
- Posterior shoulder dislocations

Radiographic Evaluation
- AP, lateral, and scapular Y views

Management
- Immobilization in sling

Disposition
- Discuss with orthopedic specialist while patient is in the ED

Surgical Neck Fracture (Proximal Humerus Fracture)

General
- Arm usually held in AD-duction
  - High incidence of neurovascular injury if arm is held in AB-duction
- Do not attempt to AD-duct the arm (may cause neurovascular damage)
- Immobilize arm in AB-duction before imaging

Associated Injuries
- Axillary nerve injury (see Chapter 14)

Radiographic Evaluation
- AP views in internal and external rotation, scapular Y view, axillary view
- Consider CT for occult fractures

Management
- Reduction if vascular compromise and emergent orthopedic consultation unavailable
- Immobilization in sling +/- swathe

Steps	Surgical Neck Reduction Technique
1	Place patient in supine or 45° upright position
2	Apply axial traction to the distal humerus
3	Medially rotate the arm across the anterior chest, then slightly flex
4	Place the other hand on the medial aspect of the humerus and attempt to manually reposition the distal fragment
5	Release traction gradually
6	Perform a complete neurovascular exam and place arm in a sling and swathe dressing

Disposition

- Discuss with orthopedic specialist while patient is in the ED
  - Displaced fractures will often require surgical management

HUMERAL SHAFT FRACTURE

General

- Fracture of the middle 1/3 of the humerus from lesser tubercle to supracondylar ridges
  - Patterns include transverse, oblique, spiral, comminuted
- Mechanism: direct or indirect trauma from a fall
- Exam: obvious deformity +/- shortening

Associated Injuries

- Other fractures including shoulder or distal humerus fractures
  - Floating elbow: concurrent ipsilateral humeral and forearm shaft fractures
- Median, radial, ulnar nerve injuries (see Chapter 14)
- Brachial artery injury
- Compartment syndrome

Radiographic Evaluation

- AP and lateral views

Management

- Immobilization in U-shaped coaptation splint +/- collar and cuff, or sling and swathe

Disposition
- Discuss with orthopedic specialist while patient is in the ED
  — Practice patterns vary regarding indications for surgical management

SCAPULAR FRACTURE

General
- Fractures classified by anatomical location
  — Scapular body is most common
- Mechanism: typically direct blow
- Exam: arm held in AD-duction, pain worse with AB-duction

Associated Injuries
- Scapular neck and body
  — Thoracic aortic injury: classic teaching but < 1% in clinical practice
  — Pneumothorax, hemothorax, rib fracture, pulmonary contusion
  — Injuries to axillary nerve (see Chapter 14), axillary artery, and brachial plexus (see Chapter 14)
- Acromion: lateral clavicular fracture, brachial plexus injury, AC joint injuries
- Glenoid neck: proximal humerus fracture, shoulder dislocation, clavicular fracture (floating shoulder)
- Glenoid rim: shoulder dislocation
- Coracoid: brachial plexus injury (see Chapter 14), AC separation, clavicular fracture

Radiographic Evaluation
- AP and scapular Y views
- Consider CT for complex fractures

Management
- Immobilization in sling
- Indications for surgical management: glenohumeral instability, displaced scapular neck fracture, open fracture, loss of rotator cuff function, displaced coracoid fracture

Disposition
- Discuss with orthopedic specialist while patient is in the ED

SHOULDER DISLOCATIONS

General
- Disarticulation of the glenohumeral joint
- Classified as anterior (~95%), posterior (~5%), or inferior (< 1%)
- Likelihood of successful reduction in ED decreases with duration of shoulder being dislocated

Associated Injuries
- Rotator cuff injuries
- Fractures
  - Risk factors include age > 40, first-time dislocation, humeral ecchymoses, traumatic mechanism
- Neurovascular injury

Anterior Shoulder Dislocation

General
- Displacement of the humeral head anterior to the glenoid fossa
  - Can be subcoracoid (90%), subclavicular, or subglenoid
  - Pseudodislocation: hemarthrosis can cause widening of the joint space, usually seen with proximal humerus fractures

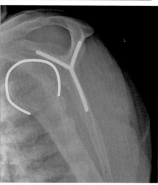

Anterior Shoulder Dislocation—Y View

- Mechanism: AB-duction and external rotation (hyper-external rotation)
- Exam: arm held at side with "squared off" shoulder (prominent acromion process), absence of humeral head directly below the acromion, inability to touch opposite shoulder with affected arm

Associated Injuries

- Subclavicular and subglenoid dislocations associated with rotator cuff tear or greater tuberosity fracture
- Hill-Sachs defect
  — Impaction of the base of the humeral head against the anterior glenoid
  — High incidence with anterior dislocations (usually when recurrent)
- Bankart lesion
  — Labrum tear +/- injury to joint capsule
  — Bony Bankart: fracture of the anteroinferior glenoid rim
- Axillary nerve injury (see Chapter 14)
- Joint capsule/ligaments injury

Radiographic Evaluation

- AP and scapular Y views
  — Consider axillary view of scapula (15° of AB-duction is sufficient) and/or Velpeau axillary view (if ambulatory) if concern for false negative Y view

Management

- Reduction and immobilization with sling +/- swathe or shoulder immobilizer
  — Younger patients may require longer immobilization (up to 3 weeks) due to higher rates of recurrence

Anterior Shoulder Dislocation Reduction Techniques

Technique	Description
Axial (In-line) Traction (supine)	• Grasp distal arm, AB-duct arm above 90° while applying traction and external rotation • If needed, increase AB-duction and apply superior force to the humeral head • An assistant can apply countertraction using a sheet around the affected shoulder, standing by the contralateral hip, and leaning backwards
Cunningham (seated)	• Grasp proximal forearm, flex elbow to 90° and AD-duct arm to abut the torso • Apply gentle inferior traction with one hand while massaging the trapezius, deltoid, and biceps muscles

External Rotation (supine)	• AD-duct arm to hug the axilla with one hand
	• Grasp wrist with other hand and flex elbow to 90°
	• Use forearm as a lever to apply gentle external rotation (reduction usually occurs between 70–110° of external rotation)
FARES (Modified Milch) (supine)	• Grasp distal forearm, apply gentle axial traction, move extended forearm though oscillating anterior/posterior movements while concurrently AB-ducting the arm
	• At 90° of AB-duction, externally rotate arm
Milch (supine or prone)	• Grasp wrist and fully AB-ducting arm above head
	• Apply gentle axial traction and external rotation
	• If needed, apply superolateral force to humeral head to push it back into the glenoid fossa
Scapular Manipulation (seated or prone)	• Assistant: facing patient, grasp wrist and apply forward traction to extend arm parallel to floor while applying countertraction with other hand at patient's clavicle, externally rotate if needed
	• Operator: stabilize scapula with one hand on the superolateral border with the other hand on the inferior angle, then rotate the inferior angle medially and superolateral border laterally with mild dorsal displacement by lifting the inferior angle
	• Prone: perform in conjunction with Stimson technique (see below)
Spaso (supine)	• Grasp wrist and lift towards ceiling while applying axial traction and external rotation
	• If needed, use other hand to apply direct pressure humeral head
Stimson Maneuver (prone)	• Arm hangs off stretcher pointing to floor with 5–10 lbs of weight secured to the wrist (may need to anchor patient to stretcher)
	• Maintain position for 15–20 minutes or successful reduction
	• If needed, can apply external rotation, forward flexion, or scapular manipulation

Traction/ Countertraction (supine)	• Elevate bed to level of assistant's hips and pass a sheet over the chest, through the axilla, under the back, and tie to assistant's waist • Assistant: leans back to provide countertraction force • Operator: grasp proximal forearm and apply axial traction with forearm flexed to 90° and arm AB-ducted to 90° (ie, elbow points to side and forearm points to ceiling) • If needed, apply slight external rotation

Note: Kocher and Hippocratic techniques are no longer recommended because of high incidence of complications.

Disposition
- ED discharge and follow-up with orthopedic specialist if successful reduction

Inferior Shoulder Dislocation (Luxatio Erecta)

General
- Displacement of the humeral head inferior to the glenoid fossa (rare)
- Mechanism: forceful hyperabduction of the arm
- Exam: affected arm held elevated with inability to AD-duct (looks like they are raising their arm to ask a question)

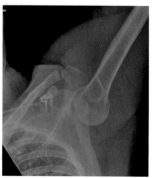

AP View

Associated Injuries
- Greater tuberosity (most common associated fracture)
- Inferior capsule (almost always) and rotator cuff (common) injuries
- Compression injuries, most often to axillary artery and brachial plexus, are common and typically resolve after reduction

Radiographic Evaluation
- AP and scapular Y views

Management
- Reduction and immobilization with sling and swathe or shoulder immobilizer

Inferior Shoulder Dislocation Reduction Techniques

	Reduction Technique 1	
Steps	First Person	Second Person
1	Grasp wrist and apply axial traction, then AD-duct the arm	Apply countertraction with a folded sheet wrapped around torso just medial to the affected shoulder

Steps	Reduction Technique 2 (Converts inferior dislocation to an anterior dislocation)
1	Stand on affected side with patient supine
2	Apply pressure to lateral mid-humerus while simultaneously pulling elbow at the medial epicondyle
3	This should convert the dislocation to an anterior (patient will be able to AD-duct arm)
4	Reduce anterior dislocation to complete reduction

Disposition
- ED discharge and follow-up with orthopedic specialist if successful reduction

Posterior Shoulder Dislocation

General
- Displacement of the humeral head posterior to the glenoid fossa
  - Includes subacromial (most common), subglenoid, and subspinous
- Most commonly missed major dislocation
- Mechanism: forceful internal rotation (eg, from seizure or electrical shock)
- Exam: arm held AD-ducted and internally rotated with limited ability to AB-duct and externally rotate

Associated Injuries

- Fracture of the humerus and with fracture of the posterior aspect of the glenoid rim
- Isolated fracture of the lesser tuberosity (assume concurrent posterior dislocation)
- Reverse Hill-Sachs deformity
  - Impaction fracture of the anteromedial humeral head from the posterior glenoid rim
- Neurovascular injury uncommon

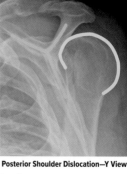

Posterior Shoulder Dislocation—Y View

Radiographic Evaluation

- AP and lateral views
  - Consider Y or axillary views if unclear
  - Rim signs: either humeral head overlapping the anterior glenoid rim or widening of the joint space (> 6 mm)
  - Lightbulb/ice cream cone sign: circular appearing humeral head due to internal rotation
- Consider CT scan for occult dislocations or evaluation of concurrent fractures

Management

- Reduction and immobilization with sling and swathe or shoulder immobilizer

Posterior Shoulder Dislocation Reduction Techniques

Steps	Reduction Technique
1	Apply axial traction to flexed and AD-ducted shoulder
2	Apply direct pressure on the posterior humeral head
3	Immobilize with sling and swathe or shoulder immobilizer

- Indications for operative treatment: lesser tuberosity displacement that doesn't reduce with shoulder reduction, articular defect > 25%, dislocation > 3 weeks

Disposition

- Discuss with orthopedic specialist while patient is in the ED

CHAPTER 6

Elbow

FRACTURES BY LOCATION

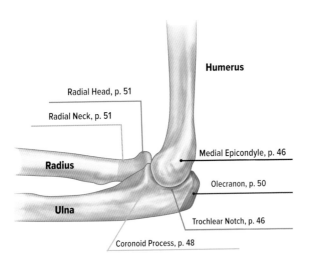

Humerus

Radial Head, p. 51

Radial Neck, p. 51

Radius

Medial Epicondyle, p. 46

Olecranon, p. 50

Ulna

Trochlear Notch, p. 46

Coronoid Process, p. 48

ELBOW IMAGING

Recommended Views
- AP: demonstrates distal humerus, proximal ulna, radius
  — Shows medial and lateral epicondyles
- Lateral: demonstrates ulna-trochlear joint, coronoid process, olecranon process
  — Anterior humeral line

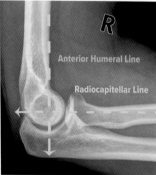

- Line drawn down the anterior surface of the humerus should intersect the middle 1/3 of the capitellum in children > age 4
- Misalignment suggests supracondylar fracture
  — Radiocapitellar line
    - Line drawn down the center of the neck of the radius should intersect the middle of the capitellum
    - Misalignment suggests radial head fracture and/or dislocation

Additional Views
- Internal (medial) oblique: visualization of medial epicondyle and coronoid process
- External (lateral) oblique: visualization of capitulum and head of radius

Views for trauma or inability to tolerate normal views
- Horizontal beam lateral: modified lateral projection that requires little to no patient movement
- Acute flexion AP: modified AP projection when the patient cannot straighten the arm
- Inferosuperior view: modified elbow projection for patients in acute flexion > 90°

Pediatric Ossification Centers for the Elbow
- When evaluating pediatric films, be aware that the joint matures at different age
- CRITOE mnemonic is helpful

	Ossification Center	Age of Ossification
C	**C**apitellum	1
R	**R**adial Head	3
I	**I**nternal (*medial*) Epicondyle	5
T	**T**rochlea	7
O	**O**lecranon	9
E	**E**xternal (*lateral*) Epicondyle	11

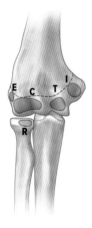
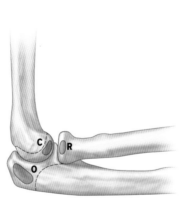

CAPITELLUM AND TROCHLEA FRACTURES

General
- Isolated fractures are very rare
  — Can see with posterior elbow dislocations
- Mechanism: FOOSH
- Exam: typically delayed presentation of swelling and pain worse with elbow flexion

Associated Injuries
- Radial head fractures
- Ulnar collateral ligament injury with capitellum fractures

Radiographic Evaluation
- AP and lateral views

Management
- Immobilization in posterior long-arm splint

Disposition
- Discuss with orthopedic specialist while patient is in the ED
  — Trochlea or large capitellum fractures almost always require surgical management

CONDYLAR FRACTURE (LATERAL AND MEDIAL)

General
- Includes both articular segment and a non-articular epicondylar segment
  — Lateral involves capitellum and lateral epicondyle (more common)
  — Medial involves trochlea and medial epicondyle (less common)
- Classified by whether lateral trochlear ridge is involved
- Mechanism
  — Lateral: posterior force applied to flexed elbow or AD-duction and hyperextension of extended elbow
  — Medial: medial force applied to flexed elbow or AB-duction of extended elbow
- Exam: pain worse with wrist flexion/extension

Associated Injuries

- None commonly seen

Radiographic Evaluation

- AP and lateral views
  - Ⓟ Comparison views if pediatric patient

Management

- Immobilization in posterior long-arm splint with forearm supinated (lateral condyle) or pronated (medial condyle)
  - Add anterior long-arm splint to above if lateral trochlear ridge involvement

Disposition

- Discuss with orthopedic specialist while patient is in the ED
  - Almost always requires surgical management

EPICONDYLAR FRACTURE (Ⓟ PEDIATRIC)

General

- Avulsion fracture of the medial epicondyle with concurrent posterior elbow dislocation most common
- Mechanism
  - Medial: posterior elbow dislocation, repetitive stress ("Little League elbow")
  - Lateral (rare): direct blow
- Exam: pain worse with pronation or elbow/wrist flexion

Associated Injuries

- Ulnar nerve injury (see Chapter 14) with medial epicondylar fractures
- Posterior elbow dislocation

Radiographic Evaluation

- AP and lateral with comparison views

Management

- Reduction (if concurrent elbow dislocation) and immobilization in posterior long-arm splint with forearm pronated (medial epicondyle) or supinated (lateral epicondyle)

Disposition

- Discuss with pediatric orthopedic specialist while patient is in the ED
  - If non-operative, follow-up with specialist in 5–7 days

CORONOID PROCESS FRACTURE

General
- Classified as non-displaced, displaced, or displaced with posterior elbow dislocation
- Mechanism: hyperextension injury when isolated, anterior force from humerus when with posterior elbow dislocation
- Exam: tenderness in the antecubital fossa

Radiographic Evaluation
- AP and lateral views
  — Consider oblique views
- Consider CT for occult fractures

Management
- Reduction (if concurrent elbow dislocation) and immobilization in posterior long-arm splint with forearm supinated

Disposition
- Discuss with orthopedic specialist while patient is in the ED
  — Displaced fractures usually require surgical management

ELBOW DISLOCATION

General
- Simple (no fractures) or complex (with fractures)
- Direction of dislocation
  — Posterior/posterolateral: most common, olecranon is dislocated posterior to humerus
  — Anterior: almost always with concurrent fractures
  — Medial and lateral: most often with concurrent anterior/posterior dislocation or fractures

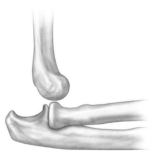

- Mechanism
  — Posterior: fall on extended AB-ducted arm
  — Anterior: blow to back of flexed elbow

- Exam
  - Posterior: elbow flexed with prominent olecranon posteriorly
  - Anterior: elbow extended, forearm supinated and appears elongated

Associated Injuries
- "Terrible Triad": posterior elbow dislocation with radial head and coronoid fractures
- Ulnar and/or medial nerve injury (see Chapter 14)
- Shoulder and/or wrist injuries
- Compartment syndrome
- Vascular injury common in anterior dislocations

Radiographic Evaluation
- AP and lateral views

Management
- Posterior dislocations: reduction and immobilization in posterior long-arm splint
- Anterior dislocations: immobilization in presenting position, discuss with orthopedic specialist prior to reduction because of high incidence of neurovascular injuries

Posterior Elbow Dislocation Reduction Techniques

Technique	Description
Kumar (supine)	• Have patient place arm across their chest with elbow at 90°
	• Grasp distal forearm with one hand while other hand grasps elbow with thumb over the olecranon and fingers over the proximal forearm
	• Apply axial traction and slowly flex elbow while pushing olecranon back into position with thumb
Leverage (supine)	• Supinate forearm and AB-duct shoulder
	• Operator places their own elbow on patient's distal arm (above antecubital fossa) and grasps wrist (or interlocks fingers with patient's fingers)
	• Apply axial traction and gradually flex patient's elbow while operator's elbow provides countertraction

Modified Stimson (prone)	• Position patient so forearm hangs towards floor with elbow at edge of the stretcher • Grasp distal forearm and apply slow continuous axial (downward traction) while the other hand manipulates the olecranon
Traction/ Countertraction (seated)	• Supinate forearm and flex elbow to ~30° • Grasp distal arm (above antecubital fossa) to stabilize and apply countertraction if needed • Grasp wrist with other hand and apply slow continuous axial traction • Can also have assistant stabilize distal forearm so operator can use other hand to manipulate the olecranon

Disposition
- If adequate reduction and no fractures: ED discharge and follow-up with orthopedic specialist
- All other cases: discuss with orthopedic specialist while patient is in the ED

OLECRANON FRACTURE

General
- All are considered intra-articular
  — Displaced if fragment separation > 2 mm
- Mechanism: direct trauma or FOOSH
- Exam: unable to extend elbow against gravity

Associated Injuries
- Ulnar nerve injury (see Chapter 14)
- Elbow dislocations
- Radial head/shaft and distal humerus fractures

Radiographic Evaluation
- AP and lateral views
  — Consider radiocapitellar views to evaluate for associated injuries

Management
- Immobilization in posterior long-arm splint with elbow flexed 50–90°

Disposition

- Discuss with orthopedic specialist while patient is in the ED
  - Displaced fractures almost always require surgical management

RADIAL HEAD/NECK FRACTURE

General

- Most common elbow fracture in adults
- Includes marginal (intra-articular), neck, and comminuted fractures
- Mechanism: FOOSH
- Exam: pain worse with supination

Associated Injuries

- Capitellum fracture
- "Terrible triad": posterior elbow dislocation with radial head and coronoid fractures
- Essex-Lopresti fracture dislocation (see p. 61)
  - Suspect if patient has wrist pain with radial head fracture

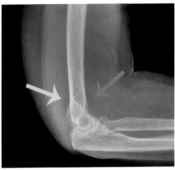

Posterior Fat Pad

- Lateral collateral ligament (LCL) and/or medial collateral ligament (MCL) injury
- Olecranon fracture
- Median nerve injury (see Chapter 14)

Radiographic Evaluation

- AP and lateral views
  - Posterior fat pad (yellow arrow) and enlarged/elevated anterior fat pad (sail sign—green arrow)
  - Evaluate radiocapitellar line (see p. 44)
  - Consider lateral oblique view for radial head fractures
- Consider CT for severely comminuted fractures

Management
- Reduction and immobilization in posterior long-arm splint
- Consider joint aspiration to reduce pain

Disposition
- Discuss with orthopedic specialist while patient is in the ED
  - Typically requires surgical management

RADIAL HEAD SUBLUXATION (🅟 PEDIATRIC)

General
- Also known as nursemaid's elbow, most often seen in children ages 2–5 years
- Mechanism: caused by longitudinal traction on an outstretched arm, resulting in subluxation of annular ligament
- Exam: arm usually held at the side with pronated forearm and slightly flexed elbow

Associated Injuries
- Associated fractures uncommon

Radiographic Evaluation
- Clinical diagnosis
  - Consider AP and lateral views if unable to reduce after 3 attempts, concern for fracture, or patient unable to move arm 15 minutes after reduction

Management
- Reduction with either hyperpronation or supination/flexion technique
  - Child will typically use arm within 10-15 minutes after a successful reduction
  - Educate parents on refraining from activities that involve pulling on affected arm

Steps	Supination/Flexion Technique	Hyperpronation Technique
1	Hold elbow while applying pressure on the radial head with thumb or forefinger	
2	Use other hand to supinate forearm then flex elbow	Keep elbow at 90° and use other hand to hyper-pronate the forearm
3	Palpable/audible "click" usually indicates successful reduction	

Disposition

- If fractured: discuss with pediatric orthopedic specialist while patient is in the ED
- Not fractured: ED discharge with follow-up as needed

SUPRACONDYLAR FRACTURE

General

- Transverse fracture of the distal humerus above the joint capsule that occurs when the diaphysis of the humerus dissociates from the condyles
  - Intercondylar fracture: supracondylar with a vertical component
  - Bimodal age distribution: kids and older adults
- Mechanism: FOOSH or fall on elbow
  - In elderly adults, can be intra-articular after a fall on flexed elbow

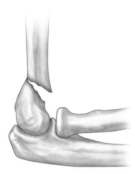

Type II Supracondylar Fracture

- Exam: impaired movement at elbow (avoid range of motion testing until displaced fracture is ruled-out)
- Classified as Gartland Type I–III

Associated Injuries

- Distal radius fracture
- Medial condyle fracture
- Floating elbow (supracondylar fracture with concurrent fractures of the ipsilateral forearm bones)
- Olecranon avulsion fracture
- Anterior interosseous, median, radial, ulnar nerve injuries (see Chapter 14)
- Brachial and/or radial artery injuries
- Compartment syndrome (concurrent nerve injury may mask symptoms)

Radiographic Evaluation

- AP and lateral views
  - Findings include posterior fat pad sign and anterior humeral line displacement

Management

- Reduction only if limb-threatening vascular compromise
- Immobilization in posterior long-arm splint (forearm positioning is controversial, so discuss with orthopedic specialist prior to splinting)

Disposition

- Discuss with orthopedic specialist while patient is in the ED
  - Almost always requires surgical management

TRANSCONDYLAR FRACTURE

General

- Transverse fracture involving both condyles within the joint capsule
  - Rare, typically seen in older patients
- Classified by position of distal humerus segment
  - Flexion: Anterior to proximal humerus
    - Posadas fracture: flexion transcondylar fracture associated with posterior dislocation of the radius or ulna
  - Extension: Posterior to proximal humerus
- Mechanism: direct blow to flexed elbow
- Exam: localized tenderness, deformity

Associated Injuries

- High risk of vascular injury

Radiographic Evaluation

- AP and lateral views

Management

- Immobilization in posterior long-arm splint in presenting position
  - Repositioning the arm can precipitate vascular injury

Disposition

- Discuss with orthopedic specialist while patient is in the ED
  - Almost always requires surgical management

CHAPTER 7

Forearm and Wrist

FRACTURES BY LOCATION

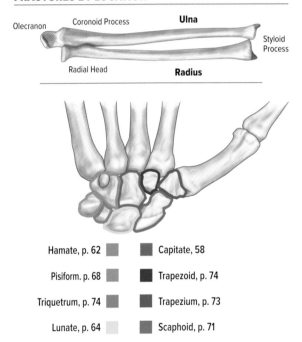

Hamate, p. 62	Capitate, 58
Pisiform. p. 68	Trapezoid, p. 74
Triquetrum, p. 74	Trapezium, p. 73
Lunate, p. 64	Scaphoid, p. 71

Distal Radius Imaging

- PA wrist view: best view to assess carpal bone joint spaces and distal radioulnar joint (DRUJ)
  — Signs of dislocation of the DRUJ
- Ulnar styloid fracture at the base
- Widening of the DRUJ space > 2 mm on AP view
- Relative shortening of the radius by > 5 mm
- Dorsal displacement of ulnar head relative to radius in lateral view
- Oblique wrist view: best for assessing trapezium-trapezoid joint
- Lateral wrist view: best for assessing alignment of radius, lunate, and capitate for suspected dislocation
- Clenched fist view: best for assessing scapholunate dissociation

HIGH-RISK FINDINGS IN DISTAL RADIUS FRACTURES

Radiographic findings on initial X-rays that are risk factors for secondary displacement (and need for surgical management) despite adequate reduction and splinting

- 20° of dorsal or volar angulation
- Displacement > 2/3 width of the shaft in either direction
- Metaphyseal comminution
- Shortening > 5 mm
- Intra-articular component
- Associated ulnar fracture
- Severe osteoporosis or osteopenia

BARTON FRACTURE

General

- Distal radial fracture with dislocation of radiocarpal joint and an intra-articular fracture involving the volar or dorsal rim
  — Volar Barton is a Smith fracture, dorsal Barton similar to a Colles

- Mechanism: FOOSH or high-energy traumas
- Exam: localized tenderness, swelling, deformity

Associated Injuries
- Carpal bone injuries
- Radial nerve injury

Radiographic Evaluation
- Forearm AP and lateral views
- Wrist PA, lateral, and oblique views
- Consider CT or MRI if severely comminuted

Management
- Reduction (if displaced) and immobilization in sugar tong splint with forearm neutral

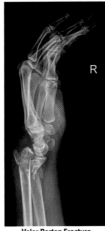

Volar Barton Fracture

Dorsal Barton Reduction Technique

Steps	First Person	Second Person
1	Hyperextend the wrist (after traction and countertraction applied)	Provide traction and countertraction at the wrist
2	Place 2 thumbs over the fragment	
3	Provide traction distally and flex the wrist	
4	Splint in sugar tong with wrist slightly extended	

Volar Barton Reduction Technique

Steps	First Person	Second Person
1	Hyperflex the wrist (after traction and countertraction applied)	Provide traction and countertraction at the wrist
2	Place 2 thumbs over the fragment	
3	Provide traction distally and extend the wrist	
4	Splint in sugar tong with wrist slightly flexed	

Disposition
- Discuss with hand specialist while patient is in the ED
  — Usually requires surgical management

CAPITATE FRACTURE

General
- Isolated fractures extremely rare
- Typically non-displaced transverse fracture
- Mechanism: direct force over the distal dorsum of the wrist or FOOSH
- Exam: pain at the dorsum of the hand over the capitate bone, and pain with axial compression of the third metacarpal

Associated Injuries
- Fractures of the radius and/or neighboring carpal bones
- Carpal bone dislocations
- Scaphocapitate fracture syndrome: proximal capitate fracture with concurrent scaphoid waist fracture

Radiographic Evaluation
- Wrist PA, lateral, and oblique (poor sensitivity)
- Consider CT for occult fractures

Management
- Confirmed or suspected fracture: Immobilization in thumb spica splint with wrist in slight dorsiflexion

Disposition
- ED discharge and follow-up with hand specialist

COLLES FRACTURE

General

- Distal radius fracture with dorsal displacement or angulation, usually extra-articular
  — Severe forces can cause intra-articular extension
- Mechanism: FOOSH or high-energy trauma
- Exam: "dinner fork" deformity

Associated Injuries

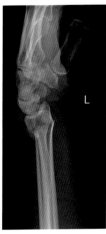

- Ulnar styloid or neck fracture (can create unstable distal radioulnar joint)
- Carpal bone fractures
- Distal radioulnar subluxation
- Scapholunate dissociation
- Ligamentous, flexor tendon, and median/ulnar nerve injuries (see Chapter 14)
- Severely comminuted fractures or fractures requiring multiple reduction attempts are at high risk for median nerve damage and acute carpal tunnel syndrome

Radiographic Evaluation

- Forearm AP and lateral views
- Wrist PA, lateral, and oblique views
- Consider CT if significant intra-articular involvement

Management

- Reduction and immobilization in sugar tong splint

Colles Fracture Reduction Techniques

Steps	First Person	Second Person
1	Flex elbow 90°	Provide traction and countertraction between fingers and elbow (can also consider finger traps with 5–10 lbs of weight suspended at the elbow)
2	Place thumbs on dorsal aspect of distal fragment and wrap fingers around wrist, then recreate force of injury by slightly extending the dorsal fracture fragment	Apply and maintain countertraction
3	Apply volar pressure to the distal fragment with thumbs and dorsal pressure to the proximal segment with fingers	
4	Immobilize in sugar tong splint with 25° of forearm pronation, 15° of palmar flexion, and 10–15° of ulnar deviation	

- Indications for surgical management: severely comminuted or displaced (> 2 mm) intra-articular fractures, dorsal displacement > 3 mm or angulation > 10° after reduction

Disposition
- Discuss with orthopedic specialist while patient is in the ED
  — If reduction is adequate or not required, can usually ED discharge and follow-up with orthopedic specialist

ESSEX-LOPRESTI FRACTURE-DISLOCATION

General
- Triad of radial head fracture, distal radioulnar joint (DRUJ) dislocation, and interosseous membrane disruption
  - Suspect if wrist pain with radial head fracture, as missed DRUJ injuries can lead to severe wrist pain +/- loss of forearm mobility
- Mechanism: usually because of high-energy forearm trauma
- Exam: pain at lateral aspect of elbow and DRUJ worse with motion of forearm/wrist

Associated Injuries
- Forearm and elbow fractures

Radiographic Evaluation
- Forearm AP and lateral views
  - Assess radiocapitellar line on lateral view (see p. 44)
- Wrist PA, lateral, and oblique views

Management
- Reduction of fracture and DRUJ dislocation and immobilization in sugar tong splint with forearm placed in full supination

Disposition
- Discuss with orthopedic specialist while patient is in the ED
  - Almost always requires surgical management

GALEAZZI FRACTURE-DISLOCATION

General
- Fracture of the middle-distal third of the radius coupled with dislocation of distal radioulnar joint (DRUJ)
  - DRUJ instability is more common with fractures > 7.5 mm from distal radial articular surface
- Mechanism: FOOSH with hyper-pronated forearm
- Exam: deformity, wrist pain with DRUJ stress and range of motion

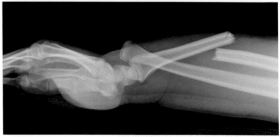

Galeazzi Fracture—Dislocation

Associated Injuries
- Compartment syndrome (See Chapter 14) if extensive soft tissue damage
- Injury to the anterior interosseous nerve (see Chapter 14)

Radiographic Evaluation
- Forearm AP and lateral views
- Wrist PA, lateral, and oblique views

Management
- Reduction and immobilization in a double sugar tong splint with forearm in moderate supination

Disposition
- Discuss with orthopedic specialist while patient is in the ED, as definitive management varies by fracture characteristic and age
  - Usually requires surgical management

HAMATE FRACTURE

General
- Distal articular surface fracture
  - Mechanism: force to flexed and ulnar deviated hand
  - Exam: pain with axial compression of 5th metacarpal
- Comminuted body fracture
  - Mechanism: direct force to dorsiflexed hand
  - Exam: pain with wrist motion

- Proximal pole articular surface fracture
  - Mechanism: direct force to dorsiflexed and ulnar deviated hand
  - Exam: pain with wrist motion
- Hook of the hamate fracture
  - Can be confused with *os hamulus proprium* (unfused hamulus), as the hook has its own ossification center and may be a normal anatomical variant in some adults
  - Mechanism: forceful compression associated with racket sports
  - Exam: tenderness over the hook (palmar surface, 1–2 cm distal and radial to pisiform) or positive hook of hamate pull test (pain with extension of 4th and 5th digits with wrist in slight ulnar deviation)

Associated Injuries
- Ulnar artery and/or nerve injuries (see Chapter 14)
- Avascular changes (low risk if early immobilization)
- Rupture of flexor digitorum profundus tendon

Radiographic Evaluation
- Wrist PA, lateral, and oblique views (low sensitivity)
  - Consider carpal tunnel or 15° reversed oblique views to assess for hook fractures
- Consider CT scan with hands in "praying position" (identifies fractures and provides comparison)

Management
- Immobilization in volar forearm or ulnar gutter splint
- Indications for surgical management: displaced fractures in patients that cannot tolerate prolonged immobilization

Disposition
- ED discharge and follow-up with hand specialist

LUNATE AND PERILUNATE DISLOCATION

General

- High-energy injuries disrupting the radius-lunate-capitate-metacarpal column articulations
  - Lunate dislocation involves volar (anterior) displacement of the lunate while the capitate remains in place
  - Perilunate dislocation involves the lunate remaining in place while the capitate dislocates and no longer articulates with the lunate
- Commonly missed on initial presentation
- Mechanism: traumatic injury to the hand with wrist extended and ulnar deviation, resulting in ligamentous injury +/- concurrent fractures
- Exam: pain worse with wrist movement

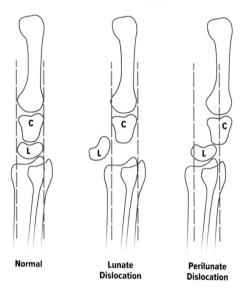

| Normal | Lunate Dislocation | Perilunate Dislocation |

Associated Injuries

- Perilunate dislocations: scaphoid fracture (common), other carpal bone fractures, radial styloid fracture
- Lunate dislocations: median nerve injury (see Chapter 14)

Radiographic Evaluation

- Wrist PA, lateral, and oblique
  - Perilunate dislocation
    - PA view: increased overlap of capitate and lunate
    - Lateral view: lunate articulates with the radius but not the capitate
  - Lunate dislocation
    - PA view: "Piece of Pie"/Triangular appearance
    - Lateral view: "Spilled teacup" appearance, lunate does not articulate with capitate or radius
- Consider CT for occult fractures

Management

- Reduction and immobilization in sugar tong or volar splint

Disposition

- Discuss with orthopedic specialist while patient is in the ED
  - Usually requires surgical management

LUNATE FRACTURE

General

- Lunate body and dorsal avulsion fractures most common
- Mechanism: hand hyperextension (dorsal avulsion fracture), axial compression (body facture)
- Exam: pain worse with axial compression of the third metacarpal

Associated Injuries

- Fractures of the radius and/or neighboring carpal bones
- Lunate/perilunate dislocations
- High risk of osteonecrosis (Kienböck's disease)

Radiographic Evaluation

- Wrist PA, lateral, and oblique views (low sensitivity)
- Consider CT for occult fractures

Management
- Immobilization in long-arm thumb spica splint with MCP joints flexed for confirmed or suspected fracture

Disposition
- ED discharge and follow-up with hand specialist

LUNATE DIE-PUNCH FRACTURE

General
- Depressed fracture of the lunate fossa of the articular surface of the distal radius
- Violent mechanism increases likelihood to be comminuted, intra-articular, and associated with other injuries
- Mechanism: high-energy compression force
- Exam: tenderness and swelling over distal radius

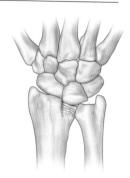

Associated Injuries
- Carpal bone injuries
- Distal radioulnar joint (DRUJ) instability

Radiographic Evaluation
- Forearm AP and lateral views
- Wrist PA, lateral, and oblique views
- Consider supinated (clenched fist) view of the wrist to evaluate for scapholunate dissociation

Management
- Immobilization in sugar tong splint

Disposition
- Discuss with orthopedic specialist while patient is in the ED
  — Usually requires surgical management

MONTEGGIA FRACTURE

General

- Displaced fractures of the proximal third of the ulnar shaft with rupture of the annular ligament leading to radial head dislocation
- More common in children (age 4–10), rare in adults
- Mechanism: fall onto an extended elbow and a hyperpronated forearm
- Exam: pain with pronation or elbow flexion/extension
  — Spontaneous radial head relocation is common

Associated Injuries

- Posterior interosseous nerve injury (see Chapter 14)
- Compartment syndrome
- Other fractures (radial head, coronoid process, olecranon)

Radiographic Evaluation

- Forearm AP/lateral and elbow AP/lateral views
  — Assess radiocapitellar line on lateral view (see p. 44)
  — Consider wrist X-rays if significant mechanism and/or pain

Management

- Immobilization in long-arm or double sugar tong splint

Disposition

- Discuss with orthopedic specialist while patient is in the ED
  — Usually requires surgical management

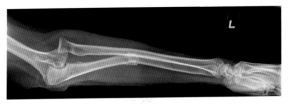

PISIFORM FRACTURE

General
- Fracture of the pisiform, a rare carpal bone fracture
- Mechanism: FOOSH
- Exam: pain at the hypothenar eminence just distal to volar crease

Associated Injuries
- High incidence of concurrent distal radius and/or other carpal bone fractures
- Ulnar nerve injury (see Chapter 14) can occur with concurrent wrist fracture or pisiform subluxation/dislocation

Radiographic Evaluation
- AP and lateral views of the carpal bones
  - Consider 30° supinated oblique and carpal tunnel views
- CT and MRI can be utilized to identify radiographically negative fractures

Management
- Immobilization in ulnar gutter or short-arm splint with ulnar deviation and 30° wrist flexion

Disposition
- Discuss with orthopedic specialist while patient is in the ED if significant concurrent and/or neurovascular injuries
  - Isolated fractures: typically ED discharge and follow-up with orthopedic specialist

RADIAL SHAFT FRACTURE (PIEDMONT FRACTURE)

General
- Isolated fracture of the radial shaft
- Mechanism: high-energy trauma or direct trauma
- Exam: localized tenderness

Associated Injuries
- High incidence of concurrent disruption of distal radioulnar joint (DRUJ)

Radiographic Evaluation
- Forearm AP and lateral views
- Wrist PA, lateral, and oblique views

Management
- Assume DRUJ instability and presence of Galeazzi fracture-dislocation
- Reduction and immobilization in a double sugar tong splint with forearm in moderate supination

Disposition
- Discuss with orthopedic specialist while patient is in the ED
  — Usually requires surgical management

RADIUS AND ULNA SHAFT FRACTURES (BOTH-BONE FOREARM FRACTURE)

General
- Concurrent shaft fractures of the radius and ulna, typically displaced and/or angulated
- Mechanism: direct or high-energy trauma (MVC most common)
- Exam: localized tenderness, deformity

Associated Injuries
- DRUJ injury
- Compartment syndrome
- Anterior and/or posterior interosseous nerve injury (see Chapter 14)

Radiographic Evaluation
- Forearm AP and lateral views
- Wrist PA, lateral, and oblique views
- Elbow AP and lateral views

Management
- Reduction and immobilization in double sugar tong splint with forearm neutral

Disposition
- Discuss with orthopedic specialist while patient is in the ED
  — Almost always requires surgical management

RADIAL STYLOID FRACTURE
(CHAUFFEUR'S OR HUTCHINSON FRACTURE)

General
- Isolated oblique fracture of the radial styloid process
- Mechanism: direct trauma or fall onto radial side
- Exam: pain in and around the anatomic snuff box

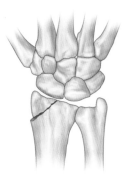

Associated Injuries
- Dorsal Barton's fracture
- Scapholunate dissociation
- Scaphoid fracture
- Trans-styloid perilunate dislocation
- Acute carpal tunnel syndrome and extensor pollicis longus (EPL) rupture

Radiographic Evaluation
- Forearm AP and lateral views
- Wrist PA, lateral, and oblique views
  - Consider supinated (clenched fist) view of the wrist to evaluate for scapholunate dissociation
- Consider CT scan if intra-articular

Management
- Immobilization in sugar tong splint

Disposition
- Discuss with orthopedic specialist while patient is in the ED
  - Usually requires surgical management due to articular involvement

SCAPHOID FRACTURE

General

- Most frequently fractured carpal bone
- Mechanism: FOOSH causing wrist hyperextension
- Exam: pain in and around anatomic snuffbox worse with axial compression of the thumb

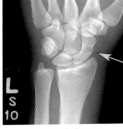

Scaphoid Waist Fracture

Associated Injuries

- Fractures of the radius and/or neighboring carpal bones
- Carpal bone dislocations
- Avascular necrosis of the proximal fracture segment

Radiographic Evaluation

- AP, lateral and scaphoid views
  — Up to 10% of initial X-rays are negative for acute fracture

Management

- Immobilization in thumb spica splint
- Consider CT, or immobilization with repeat X-rays in 7–10 days, for occult fractures

Disposition

- ED discharge and follow-up with orthopedic specialist

SMITH FRACTURE (REVERSE COLLES FRACTURE)

General

- Distal radius fracture with volar displacement or angulation
  - Distal radioulnar joint involvement is rare
  - More likely to be unstable than Colles fracture
- Mechanism: direct blow to dorsum of wrist or fall onto dorsum of hand resulting in extreme palmar flexion
- Exam: "garden spade deformity"

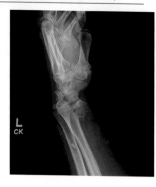

Associated Injuries

- Radial and median nerve injuries (see Chapter 14)
- Carpal fractures or dislocations (uncommon)

Radiographic Evaluation

- Forearm AP and lateral views
- Wrist PA, lateral, and oblique views

Management

- Reduction and immobilization in sugar tong splint with forearm supination and wrist neutral

Smith Fracture Reduction Technique

Steps	First Person	Second Person
1	Flex elbow 90°	Provide traction and countertraction between fingers and elbow (can also consider finger traps with 5–10 lbs of weight suspended at the elbow)
2	Flex wrist to disimpact fragments	Apply and maintain countertraction
3	Apply dorsal pressure to distal fragments	
4	Immobilize in sugar tong splint with forearm supination and wrist in neutral position	

- Indications for surgical management: open fractures, intra-articular fractures, significantly displaced or comminuted fractures, neurovascular injury

Disposition
- Discuss with orthopedic specialist while patient is in the ED
  — Almost always requires surgical management

TRAPEZIUM FRACTURE

General
- Isolated fractures are rare
- Categorized as vertical fractures, comminuted fracture, and avulsion fractures
- Mechanism: blow to AD-ducted thumb or FOOSH
- Exam: tenderness at base of thenar eminence, pain worse with thumb movement or axial compression, pain or weakness with pinching movements

Associated Injuries
- First metacarpal fracture/dislocation
- Distal radial fracture
- Flexor carpi radialis
- Radial artery injury

Radiographic Evaluation
- AP, lateral and oblique views (poor sensitivity)
  — Avulsion fractures best seen on carpal tunnel view
- Consider CT for occult fractures

Management
- Immobilization in thumb spica splint for confirmed or suspected fractures

Disposition
- ED discharge and follow-up with hand specialist

TRAPEZOID FRACTURE

General
- Dorsal dislocation much more common than fracture
- Mechanism: crush injuries
- Exam: tenderness along dorsal wrist proximal to the 2nd metacarpal base

Associated Injuries
- Other carpal/metacarpal bone fractures/dislocations
- High risk of avascular necrosis

Radiographic Evaluation
- AP, lateral and oblique views (poor sensitivity)
- Consider CT for occult fractures

Management
- Immobilization in thumb spica splint for all confirmed or suspected fractures

Disposition
- ED discharge and follow-up with hand specialist

TRIQUETRUM FRACTURE

General
- Second most commonly fractured carpal bone
- Categorized as dorsal avulsion fractures (most common) and transverse body fractures
- Mechanism: FOOSH
- Exam: dorsal pain and swelling over ulnar aspect of wrist

Associated Injuries

- Ulnar nerve and artery injury at Guyon's canal
- Perilunate dislocation with transverse fractures
- Radius or ulna fractures

Radiographic Evaluation

- AP, lateral, and oblique views (poor sensitivity)
  - Dorsal avulsion fractures best seen lateral view as a small fragment dorsal to proximal carpal row ("pooping duck" sign)
- Consider CT for occult fractures

Management

- Immobilization in volar splint with wrist in slight extension

Disposition

- Discharge and follow-up with orthopedic specialist

ULNAR SHAFT FRACTURE

General

- Classified as non-displaced, displaced (> 5 mm), and fracture-dislocation (Monteggia; see p. 67)
  - Nightstick fracture is isolated ulnar shaft fracture, usually from direct blow to forearm
- Mechanism: direct impact, classically while using arm to protect self
- Exam: localized tenderness

Associated Injuries

- Displaced ulnar fractures are associated with radial head dislocations (Monteggia fracture-dislocation) and/or radius fractures

Radiographic Evaluation

- Forearm AP and lateral views
- Elbow AP and lateral views
  - Assess radiocapitellar line on lateral view (see p. 44)

Management

- Immobilization in long-arm splint
- Indications for surgical management: < 50% apposition, > 10% angulation, proximal fractures, concurrent radial head dislocation, injury to distal or proximal radioulnar joints

Disposition
- Non-displaced fractures: ED discharge and follow-up with orthopedic specialist
- All other cases: discuss with orthopedic specialist while patient is in the ED

CHAPTER 8

Hand

FRACTURES BY LOCATION

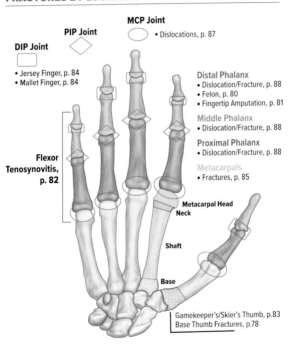

MCP Joint
• Dislocations, p. 87

PIP Joint

DIP Joint
• Jersey Finger, p. 84
• Mallet Finger, p. 84

Distal Phalanx
• Dislocation/Fracture, p. 88
• Felon, p. 80
• Fingertip Amputation, p. 81

Middle Phalanx
• Dislocation/Fracture, p. 88

Proximal Phalanx
• Dislocation/Fracture, p. 88

Metacarpals
• Fractures, p. 85

Flexor Tenosynovitis, p. 82

Metacarpal Head
Neck

Shaft

Base

Gamekeeper's/Skier's Thumb, p.83
Base Thumb Fractures, p.78

BASE OF THUMB FRACTURE

General

- Base of thumb metacarpal fractures
  - Bennett fracture: intra-articular fracture with associated subluxation or dislocation of the carpometacarpal (CMC) joint
  - Rolando fracture: comminuted intra-articular fracture through the base of the first metacarpal
  - Extra-articular fractures
- Mechanism: partially flexed thumb receives axial load ("jamming thumb")
- Exam: pain at base of the thumb worse with motion at MCP/CMC joints

Associated Injuries

- Ligamentous injury

Radiographic Evaluation

- AP, lateral, and oblique views of hand
  - Bennett fracture best seen with hyper-pronated thumb view

Management

- Immobilization in thumb spica splint
- Extra-articular fractures with angulation > 30° require reduction
- Spiral fractures often require surgical management

Disposition

- Discuss with hand specialist while patient is in the ED

EXTENSOR TENDON INJURY

General
- Injuries to tendons coursing over dorsal aspect of the hand
- Classified by zones (see table)
- Exam: normal motor function with up to 90% tendon tear, pain along the course of a tendon during resistance testing suggests a partial laceration even if strength appears adequate

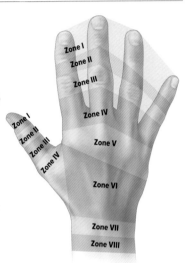

Associated Injuries
- Bony avulsion fractures

Radiographic Evaluation
- AP and lateral views of digit to evaluate for bony avulsion

Management
- Immobilization

Extensor Tendon Immobilization Techniques

Zone	Location of tendon injury	Immobilization Technique
I	Distal phalanx	Dorsal finger splint with DIP in extension
II	Middle phalanx or proximal phalanx of thumb	
III	PIP joint or MCP of thumb	Gutter or thumb spica splint with wrist in 30° of extension, MCP flexed 15–30°, and PIP neutral
IV	Proximal phalanx or base of thumb	Volar splint or thumb spica splint
V	MCP joint	Gutter or thumb spica splint with wrist in 45° of extension and MCP neutral
VI	Dorsum of hand	Gutter or thumb spica splint with wrist in 30° of extension and MCP neutral
VII	Carpal bones	Volar or thumb spica splint with wrist in 20° of extension and MCP neutral
VIII	Distal forearm	

Disposition

- Discuss with hand specialist while patient is in the ED
  — Usually requires surgical management

FELON

General

- Subcutaneous infection and abscess of the pulp of the distal fingertip
- Causative organisms include *S. aureus* and *Streptococcus* spp.
  — Consider coverage for *Eikenella* in diabetic patients who bite their nails
  — Consult *EMRA Antibiotic Guide* for current guidance

Associated Injuries

- Cellulitis, flexor tenosynovitis, septic arthritis, osteomyelitis, finger compartment syndrome with digital tip necrosis

Radiographic Evaluation
- AP and lateral views to evaluate for foreign body, subcutaneous gas, evidence of osteomyelitis
- Consider POCUS for wooden foreign bodies

Management
- Incision, drainage, and debridement
  - Surgical management may be required for deep and/or complex infections
  - Volar longitudinal incision for superficial felon, presence of foreign body, or visible drainage
  - High-lateral incision for deep felon without drainage or foreign body
- Incision on non-pressure bearing side of pulp: ulnar side of digits 2–4, radial side of digits 1 and 5
- Immobilization in finger splint
- Antibiotics, consider culturing high-risk patients

Disposition
- Discuss with hand specialist while patient is in the ED
  - May require admission for IV antibiotics +/- surgical management

FINGERTIP AMPUTATION

General
- Amputation of fingertip distal to insertion of flexor or extensor tendons
- Classification based on bony involvement or not
- Amputated tip is viable for up to 8 hours if warm or 30 hours if cold

Associated Injuries
- Injuries to the nail bed, bone, soft tissue

Radiographic Evaluation
- AP and lateral views to evaluate for bony involvement, fractures, complex dislocations

Management

- Clean wound, cover exposed bone with soft tissue, and place nonadherent dressing
  — Skin grafting indicated for areas > 1–1.5 cm
  — Operative intervention required if exposed bone or tendon, or tissue loss > 2 cm
- Antibiotics only indicated in grossly contaminated wounds
- Consider reimplantation in children, injury to the thumb, or single digit amputation proximal to the flexor digitorum superficialis
  — Relative contraindications: multiple levels of injury to the amputated part, prolonged ischemia (> 24 hours), significant comorbidities (eg, smoking history, peripheral vascular disease)

Disposition

- If reimplantation is possible or closure appears complicated: discuss with hand specialist while patient is in the ED
- All other cases: ED discharge and follow-up with hand specialist

FLEXOR TENOSYNOVITIS

General

- Acute infection within the flexor tendon synovial sheath usually obtained from penetrating trauma or direct spread from felon, septic joint, or deep space infection
- Exam: pain and swelling to the palmar aspect of the digit along with the Kanavel signs:
  1. Tenderness over the tendon sheath
  2. Severe pain with passive extension
  3. Flexed position
  4. Fusiform swelling

Associated Injuries

- Missed flexor tenosynovitis can lead to adhesions, tendon necrosis, extension into adjoining deep spaces

Radiographic Evaluation

- Consider if concern for foreign object

Management

- Hand immobilization
- Surgical management may be required for deep and/or complex infections
  - Nonoperative if early presentation and signs of improvement within 24 hours
  - Incision and drainage with culture specific antibiotics if no improvement in 24 hours

Disposition

- Discuss with hand specialist while patient is in the ED
  - May require admission for IV antibiotics

GAMEKEEPER'S/SKIER'S THUMB INJURY

General

- Injury to the ulnar collateral ligament of the thumb
- Mechanism: forced AB-duction and hyperextension of thumb MCP joint usually associated with a ski pole or athletic injury
- Exam: instability with valgus stress, especially while thumb is flexed to 30–45°, weakened pinch grip

Associated Injuries

- Avulsion or condylar fracture surrounding MCP
- Capsule or other ligamentous injury

Radiographic Evaluation

- Hand AP, lateral, and oblique views
  - Consider hyper-pronated thumb view if concern for concurrent Bennett fracture

Management

- Immobilization in thumb spica splint

Disposition

- ED discharge and follow-up with hand specialist

JERSEY FINGER

General
- Rupture of the flexor digitorum profundus tendon from distal attachment on distal phalanx
- Commonly missed by athletes as a "jammed" or sprained finger
- Mechanism: flexed DIP suddenly extended, common in contact sports
- Exam: inability to actively flex DIP joint
- Classified by Leddy and Packer Type I–IV (based on degree of tendon retraction)

Associated Injuries
- Avulsion or articular fractures
- Dorsal subluxation of distal phalanx

Radiographic Evaluation
- AP, lateral, and oblique views
- POCUS can identify tendon rupture

Management
- Immobilization in dorsal splint with 30° wrist flexion, 70° MCP flexion, 30° PIP/DIP flexion

Disposition
- Discuss with hand specialist while patient is in the ED
  — Almost always requires surgical management, usually within 1 week

MALLET FINGER

General
- Zone I extensor tendon injury to the extensor digitorum tendon at the DIP joint, 3rd and 4th digits are most common
- Mechanism: direct blow to tip of finger, causing forced flexion of the DIP
- Exam: inability to actively extend DIP, positive extensor lag, deformity (swan-neck deformity may be seen with central slip involvement)

- Seymour-type metaphyseal fracture (usually pediatric) can be mistaken for mallet finger

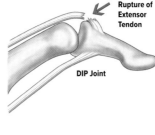

Rupture of Extensor Tendon

DIP Joint

  - Fracture between intact tendon attachments: extensor tendon posteriorly and flexor digitorum profundus tendon anteriorly
  - X-ray will differentiate metaphyseal fracture from possible tendon avulsion injury
- Classified as Doyle Type 1–4

Associated Injuries
- Avulsion and articular fractures
- Volar subluxation of DIP

Radiographic Evaluation
- AP, lateral, and oblique views

Management
- Immobilize in mallet finger splint
- Indications for surgical management: volar subluxation of distal phalanx, > 30% articular surface involved, inability to achieve full passive extension, full laceration of the tendon

Disposition
- ED discharge and follow-up with hand specialist

METACARPAL FRACTURE

General
- Classification based on location: head, neck, and shaft
  - Boxer's fracture is a metacarpal neck fracture of the 5th digit
  - 1st metacarpal fractures include extra-articular, intra-articular, and sesamoid bone
- Mechanism: direct trauma or axial loading
- Exam: localized tenderness, deformity, malrotation of digit

Associated Injuries

- CMC joint dislocation often accompanies metacarpal fractures and are often missed at initial presentation
- Rotational component maybe present and generate significant functional deficit

Radiographic Evaluation

- AP, lateral, and oblique views
- Consider CT for occult injuries, multiple CMC dislocations, complex fractures

Management

- Reduction if needed (see table) and immobilization
  - 1st metacarpal: thumb spica
  - 2nd–5th metacarpal head fractures: volar splint
  - 2nd and 3rd metacarpal neck/shaft/base: radial gutter splint
  - 4th and 5th metacarpal neck/shaft/base: ulnar gutter splint

Location	Acceptable Shaft Angulation	Acceptable Shaft Shortening (mm)	Acceptable Neck Angulation
2nd and 3rd metacarpals	10–20°	2–5	10–15°
4th metacarpal	30°	2–5	30–40°
5th metacarpal	40°	2–5	50–60°

Disposition

- Thumb fractures: discuss with orthopedic specialist while patient is in the ED

- All other cases: ED discharge and follow-up with hand specialist

METACARPOPHALANGEAL DISLOCATION

General
- Dorsal dislocation is the most common, volar is rare
- Classification based on involvement of volar plate (fibrocartilaginous structure that connects the base of the proximal phalanx to the head of the metacarpal head)
  - Simple: articulating surfaces remain in contact and volar plate and/or sesamoids are not interposed between dislocated bones
  - Complex: volar plate and/or sesamoids are interposed between dislocated bones
- Mechanism: hyperextension of MCP
- Exam: pain worse with movement at MCP joint

Associated Injuries
- Metacarpal and phalanx fractures

Radiographic Evaluation
- AP, lateral, and oblique views
  - Dislocation best seen on lateral view
  - Joint space widening and/or sesamoid bone in joint space suggest complex dislocation

Management
- Reduction of simple dislocations by hyperextension of MCP joint, then dorsal pressure to base of proximal phalanx
  - Complex dislocations almost always require surgical management
- Thumb MCP: immobilization in thumb spica splint with MCP in 20° of flexion
- Digits 2–5 immobilization in finger splint with MCP in 60° of flexion

Disposition
- Complex dislocation: discuss case with hand specialist while patient is in the ED

- All other cases: ED discharge and follow-up with hand specialist

PHALANX DISLOCATIONS/FRACTURES

General
- Proximal phalanx deformities often present with volar angulation
- Middle phalanx deformities can present with dorsal or volar angulation
- Distal phalanx fractures are the most common fractures of the hand
- Mechanism: direct trauma (sports, machinery, falls are all common)
- Exam: localized tenderness, deformity, scissoring digits if rotational component present

Associated Injuries
- Nail bed injuries (distal phalanx fractures)

Radiographic Evaluation
- Finger PA, lateral, and oblique views
  - Buckle fractures of the proximal metaphysis are commonly missed
- Hand views to rule out associated fractures

Management
- Reduction (if needed) and immobilization
  - 1st phalanx: thumb spica
  - 2nd and 3rd middle/proximal phalanx: radial gutter splint
  - 4th and 5th middle/proximal phalanx: ulnar gutter splint
  - 2nd–5th distal phalanx: finger splint
  - Consider finger splint or dynamic splinting (buddy taping) for nondisplaced middle phalanx fractures
- Indications for surgical management: irreducible or unstable fractures, displaced intra-articular fractures

Disposition
- ED discharge and follow-up with hand specialist

CHAPTER 9

Pelvis and Femur

FRACTURES BY LOCATION

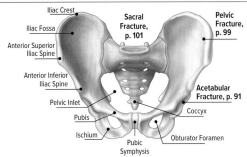

Iliac Crest

Iliac Fossa

Anterior Superior Iliac Spine

Anterior Inferior Iliac Spine

Pelvic Inlet

Pubis

Ischium

Sacral Fracture, p. 101

Pelvic Fracture, p. 99

Acetabular Fracture, p. 91

Coccyx

Obturator Foramen

Pubic Symphysis

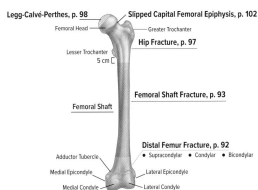

Legg-Calvé-Perthes, p. 98

Femoral Head

Slipped Capital Femoral Epiphysis, p. 102

Greater Trochanter

Hip Fracture, p. 97

Lesser Trochanter

5 cm

Femoral Shaft Fracture, p. 93

Femoral Shaft

Distal Femur Fracture, p. 92
- Supracondylar • Condylar • Bicondylar

Adductor Tubercle

Medial Epicondyle

Medial Condyle

Lateral Epicondyle

Lateral Condyle

Pelvic Imaging

- AP pelvis: evaluate for disruption, asymmetry of pelvic ring
- Inlet view: best view to assess AP displacement or SI widening
- Outlet view: best view to assess vertical displacement, sacral fractures
- Judet view: best view to assess for acetabular fractures
- CT: better evaluation of pelvic ring, acetabulum, and posterior injuries
- MRI: evaluate for spinal injury based on exam

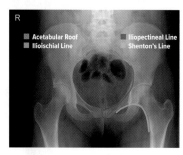

R

Acetabular Roof
Ilioischial Line
Iliopectineal Line
Shenton's Line

Pelvic Ring Injury Patterns

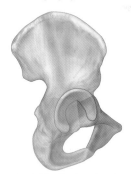

Anterior/iliopubic column (brown) injuries result when hip is externally rotated

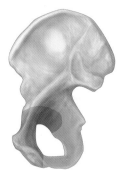

Posterior/ilioichial column (purple) injuries result when hip is internally rotated

ACETABULAR FRACTURE

General
- Fracture of the acetabulum, usually posterior wall
- Can disrupt articular surface
- Mechanism: high-energy trauma (MVC/MVA/pedestrian struck)
- Exam: hip pain and inability to bear weight

Associated Injuries
- Hip dislocation
- Spine injuries
- Sciatic nerve injury (see Chapter 14)
- Pelvic vascular injury
- Other traumatic injuries (chest, abdomen, genitourinary, etc.)

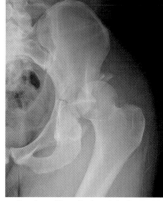

Superior and Posterior Acetabular Fracture with Hip Dislocation

Radiographic Evaluation
- AP pelvis views, Judet views
- CT after initial plain film (ideal modality)
  — If femoro-acetabular dislocation on X-ray, reduce the hip before CT imaging

Management
- Concurrent hip dislocation requires immediate reduction
- Weight bearing based on fracture type/location
- Indications for operative treatment
  — Displacement of the fracture fragment or fracture instability
  — Presence of associated fracture/dislocation

Disposition
- Discuss with orthopedic specialist while patient is in the ED

APOPHYSEAL AVULSION FRACTURE

General
- Fracture at tendon insertion site
  - Iliac crest: anterior abdominal wall muscles
  - Anterior superior iliac spine: tensor fascia lata and sartorius
  - Anterior inferior iliac spine: straight head of rectus femoris
  - Greater trochanter: gluteus medius and gluteus minimus
  - Lesser trochanter: iliopsoas muscle
  - Ischial tuberosity: hamstring muscles
  - Body and inferior ramus of pubis: thigh adductors and gracilis
- More commonly seen in athletes, especially older children/teenagers before the physis closes
- In adults, without history of trauma, avulsion fractures should be considered pathologic until proven otherwise
- Mechanism: sudden, forceful muscular contraction or excessive stretch
- Exam: pain over the avulsed area worse with passive stretch or contraction of the avulsing muscle

Associated Injuries
- Neuropathies from localized swelling (uncommon)

Radiographic Evaluation
- AP and lateral views

Management
- Conservative management
- May require surgical management if > 2 cm displacement

Disposition
- ED discharge and follow-up with orthopedic specialist

DISTAL FEMUR FRACTURE

General
- Fractures distal to the femoral shaft, which include:
  - Supracondylar/extra-articular
  - Condylar/partial articular
  - Bicondylar/complete articular

- Mechanism: high-energy trauma (younger patients), low-energy falls (older adults)
- Exam: pain/swelling/deformity at distal thigh

Associated Injuries
- Popliteal injury if significant displacement

Radiographic Evaluation
- AP and lateral views
- CTA if diminished pulses after reduction

Management
- Reduction and immobilization in posterior long-leg splint, non-weight bearing

Disposition
- Discuss with orthopedic specialist while patient is in the ED
  — Almost always requires surgical management

FEMORAL SHAFT FRACTURE

General
- Fractures involving the shaft of the femur which begins 5 cm distal to the lesser trochanter and end 6–8 cm proximal to the adductor tubercle
- Mechanism: most commonly MVC or penetrating trauma, also seen in falls in the elderly and non-accidental trauma in children
- Exam: tense/swollen/tender thigh, possible leg shortening

Associated Injuries
- Ipsilateral femoral neck fracture
- Femoral artery injury
- Sciatic, tibial, or peroneal nerve injuries (see Chapter 14) are rare
- Due to high force involved, often associated with other life-threatening injuries

Radiographic Evaluation
- AP and lateral views
  — Consider pelvis and knee X-rays (high incidence of concurrent injuries)

Management

- Immediate reduction and orthopedic consultation if signs of neurovascular injury
- Immobilization in traction splint unless concurrent fracture/ dislocation of the ipsilateral hip, knee, or ankle

Disposition

- Discuss with orthopedic specialist while patient is in the ED
  — Almost always requires surgical management

HIP DISLOCATION

General

- Displacement of the femoral head from the acetabulum
  — Simple: without associated proximal femur or acetabular fracture
  — Complex: with associated proximal femur or acetabular fracture
- Displacement can be posterior (most common) or anterior
  — Anterior dislocation can be inferior (obturator) or superior (pubic or iliac)
- Mechanism: high-energy trauma
- Exam
  — Posterior: leg held in AD-duction and internal rotation
  — Anterior: leg held in AB-duction and external rotation
- Dislocation of a non-native hip is similar to native hips
  — If recent hip replacement (< 2 weeks), discuss with orthopedic specialist before reducing

Associated Injuries

- Femur, knee, acetabular fractures
- Ligamentous injury
- Vascular injury/avascular necrosis
  — The longer the hip is dislocated, the higher the risk of avascular necrosis
- Femoral/sciatic nerve injury (see Chapter 14)

Radiographic Evaluation

- AP and lateral views
- Consider CT for occult fractures

Management

- Reduction within 6 hours and immobilization in knee immobilizer, protected weight bearing
  - Ipsilateral femur fracture is a relative contraindication for reduction
  - All techniques benefit from having an assistant stabilize the pelvis
  - Anterior dislocation reduction techniques include Allis, Bigelow, and Stimson with the following modifications:
    - Superior dislocations require hyperextension and in-line traction
    - Inferior dislocations require flexion, AD-duction, and external rotation followed by axial traction

Hip Dislocation Reduction Techniques

Technique	Description
Allis maneuver (Supine)	• Stand on affected side, grasp proximal leg, and flex knee to 90° • Apply axial traction while flexing the hip • Can apply internal/external rotation and/or AB-duction/AD-duction if needed
Bigelow maneuver (Supine)	• Stand on affected side, grasp distal tibia with one hand, and place opposite forearm under the knee • Flex hip to 90° and apply axial traction while AB-ducting, externally rotating, and extending the hip
Captain Morgan maneuver (Supine)	• Stand on affected side, flex hip and knee to 90° • Operator places their foot on the bed and their knee under the patient's knee • Grasp ankle and apply downward traction while operator plantarflexes to apply upward force at the knee • Can apply internal/external rotation and/or AB-duction/AD-duction if needed • Can use backboard to secure pelvis to bed for stability

Technique	Description
Stimson gravity maneuver (Prone)	• Patient positioned with waist at edge of bed and knees off stretcher with hips flexed to 90° • Grasp ankle with one hand and flex knee to 90° while other hand applies downward force on the proximal posterior leg • Apply internal and external rotation using hand holding ankle • Operator can also use their knee to generate downward force • Caution must be taken to ensure the patient is safely secured on the bed and their airway is protected with positioning and sedation
Tulsa technique/ Rochester method/Whistler technique (Supine, knees flexed)	• Stand on affected side, operator places their arm under patient's knee, and grasps the opposite knee • Grasp ankle with other hand and apply downward force to flex knee • Traction is maintained with arm under knee • Can apply internal and external hip rotation with hand holding ankle
Waddell technique (Supine)	• Assistant stabilizes the pelvis on affected side • Operator squats on bed, straddling patient's leg • Operator drapes patient's over forearm, stabilizing by placing elbow on one knee and hand the other knee • Operator flexes patient's knee and hip to 90° then leans backwards to generate traction (AD-duction and internal rotation can be applied with leaning and rotating) • Operator's free hand can be used to push off the assistant

Technique	Description
Other techniques	• East Baltimore lift • Flexion adduction method • Foot-fulcrum maneuver • Howard maneuver • Lateral traction method • Lefkowitz maneuver • Piggyback method • Skoff maneuver • Traction/countertraction

Disposition

- Discuss with orthopedic specialist while patient is in the ED if non-native hip dislocation, associated fractures or retained fragments, or unsuccessful reduction

HIP FRACTURE

General

- Any fracture of the proximal femur, within 5 cm of lesser trochanter, and includes:
  — Femoral head: rare, usually associated with dislocation
  — Femoral neck: includes area between femoral head and greater trochanter
  — Intertrochanteric: includes area between greater and lesser trochanter
  — Subtrochanteric: includes area 5 cm distal to lesser trochanter
- Mechanism: fall or direct trauma
- Exam: pain with active/passive range of motion, leg may be shortened and externally rotated

Associated Injuries

- Acetabular fracture, hip dislocation, femoral shaft fracture
- Sciatic nerve injury (see Chapter 14)

Radiographic Evaluation
- AP view of the hip/pelvis
- Consider MRI for occult fractures (more sensitive than CT for early detection of hip fractures)

Management
- Immobilization, non-weight bearing

Disposition
- Discuss with orthopedic specialist while patient is in the ED
  — Almost always requires surgical management

LEGG-CALVÉ-PERTHES DISEASE (Ⓟ PEDIATRIC)

General
- Avascular necrosis of the proximal femoral epiphysis, can be bilateral
- Most commonly seen in children between 4–8 years old
- Exam: typically limping, pain, limited range of motion

Associated Injuries
- No commonly associated injuries

Radiographic Evaluation
- AP pelvis and frog leg lateral views
  — Frog leg view is best view for detecting early findings in the anterior femoral epiphysis
- Consider MRI for occult injury

Management
- Conservative management, non-weight bearing or limited weight bearing

Disposition
- Discuss with pediatric orthopedic specialist while patient is in the ED
  — May require surgical management

PELVIC FRACTURE

General
- Disruption of pelvic ring from trauma
- Exam
  - Pelvic stability or instability appreciated with gentle compression/distraction of each iliac crest, performed only once
  - Consider rectal +/- vaginal speculum exam to evaluate for open fracture with rectal/vaginal perforation
- Young Burgess classification
  - Anteroposterior Compression Types I–III (open book): progressive ligament disruption of pubis symphysis then anterior SI joint then posterior SI joint

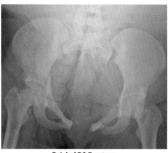

Pelvis APC Fracture

  - Lateral Compression Types I–III: progression from transverse pubic rami fractures then ilium fracture or SI joint disruption then contralateral fractures leading to external rotation of the contralateral hemipelvis

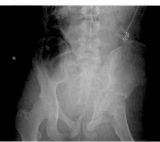

Pelvis LC Fracture

— Vertical Shear (Malgaigne fracture): requires 2 ipsilateral vertical pelvic ring injuries (one from anterior column and one from posterior column) resulting in vertical displacement of a hemipelvis

Associated Injuries
- Long bone fractures
- Lumbosacral plexus injury (see Chapter 14)
- Vascular injuries (iliac arteries and branches), hemorrhage, shock
- Abdominal injury/spine fractures
- GU injuries (bladder, urethra, perineum)

Radiographic Evaluation
- AP pelvis, inlet/outlet
- CT (ideal modality)

Management
- Unstable pelvis: pelvic binder placed over greater trochanters
  — Reduction of pelvis volume can decrease bleeding in AP/vertical shear injuries
  — May worsen lateral compression injuries

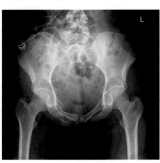

Pelvis VS Fracture

- Isolated iliac wing (Duverney's fracture): conservative management
- Consider retrograde urethrogram before Foley insertion if:
  — Blood at the urethral meatus, or gross hematuria
  — Difficulty/inability to void
  — Scrotal or penile hematoma
  — High riding or freely mobile prostate on digital rectal exam
  — Displaced fracture of pubic rami
  — Pelvic hematoma

Disposition
- Discuss with orthopedic specialist while patient is in the ED
  — Almost always requires surgical management

SACRAL FRACTURE

General
- Fracture of the sacral bone typically parallel to spine
  - Transverse or U-shaped types are associated with higher incidence of nerve injury
- Denis Classification System (see image)
  - Zone 1: fracture located lateral to foramina
  - Zone 2: fracture into foramina
  - Zone 3: fracture located medial to foramina
- Mechanism: high-energy trauma
- Exam: localized tenderness

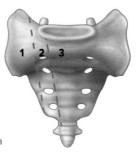

Associated Injuries
- High incidence of neurologic injury (zone 3 > 2 > 1)
  - Urinary/rectal/sexual dysfunction
- Pelvic ring disruption

Radiographic Evaluation
- AP pelvis views, inlet/outlet views (poor sensitivity)
- CT (ideal modality)
- Consider MRI if neurologic injuries

Management
- Protected weight bearing if neurologically intact and < 1 cm displaced
- Indications for surgical management include:
  - 1 cm displaced
  - Sacroiliac dislocation
  - Neurovascular injury

Disposition
- Discuss with orthopedic specialist while patient is in the ED
  - May require surgical management

General

- Slippage of metaphysis anteriorly and superiorly relative to epiphysis (SH I fracture), may be bilateral

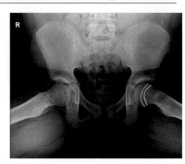

  — Commonly children 10–16 years old, often obese, may have endocrine disorder
- Mechanism: chronic shearing forces applied to femoral head exceed strength of capital femoral physis, less commonly from acute trauma
- Exam: may present as inability to walk or bear weight on the affected leg with external rotation and leg length discrepancy (affected leg shortened)

Associated Injuries

- Avascular necrosis

Radiographic Evaluation

- AP hip/pelvis and frog leg lateral views of both hips
- Consider MRI for occult fractures

Management

- Non-weight bearing

Disposition

- Discuss with pediatric orthopedic specialist while patient is in the ED
  — Usually requires surgical management

CHAPTER 10

Knee and Leg

FRACTURES BY LOCATION

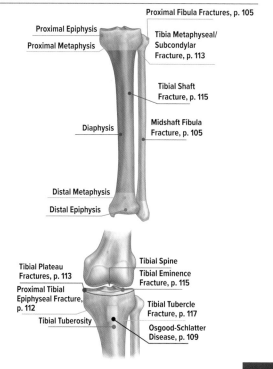

Proximal Fibula Fractures, p. 105

Proximal Epiphysis

Tibia Metaphyseal/
Subcondylar
Fracture, p. 113

Proximal Metaphysis

Tibial Shaft
Fracture, p. 115

Midshaft Fibula
Fracture, p. 105

Diaphysis

Distal Metaphysis

Distal Epiphysis

Tibial Plateau
Fractures, p. 113

Tibial Spine

Tibial Eminence
Fracture, p. 115

Proximal Tibial
Epiphyseal Fracture,
p. 112

Tibial Tubercle
Fracture, p. 117

Tibial Tuberosity

Osgood-Schlatter
Disease, p. 109

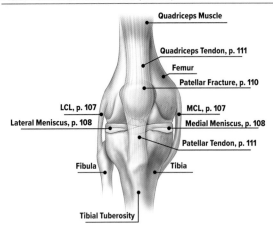

Quadriceps Muscle

Quadriceps Tendon, p. 111

Femur

Patellar Fracture, p. 110

LCL, p. 107

MCL, p. 107

Lateral Meniscus, p. 108

Medial Meniscus, p. 108

Patellar Tendon, p. 111

Fibula

Tibia

Tibial Tuberosity

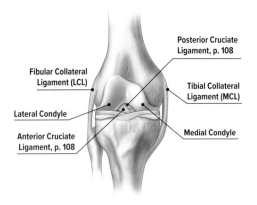

Posterior Cruciate Ligament, p. 108

Fibular Collateral Ligament (LCL)

Tibial Collateral Ligament (MCL)

Lateral Condyle

Anterior Cruciate Ligament, p. 108

Medial Condyle

Ottawa Knee Rules
- Decision-making tool to help determine need for radiographic evaluation; high sensitivity yet low specificity for clinically significant knee fractures
- Obtain imaging in patients with:
  - Age > 55
  - Isolated tenderness to palpation of patella
  - Tenderness to palpation at fibular head
  - Unable to flex knee to 90°
  - Unable to bear weight both in ED & immediately after incident (limping counts as weight bearing)

FIBULA FRACTURE (MIDSHAFT)

General
- Isolated fibular shaft fractures are uncommon
- Mechanism: direct trauma over lateral aspect of leg
- Exam: pain worse with foot eversion

Associated Injuries
- Tibia fracture
- Maisonneuve fracture

Radiographic Evaluation
- AP and lateral views

Management
- Immobilization in posterior short-leg splint (for comfort)
- Weight bearing as tolerated with crutches

Disposition
- ED discharge and follow-up with orthopedic specialist

FIBULA FRACTURE (PROXIMAL)

General
- High incidence of concurrent knee and/or ankle injuries (eg, Maisonneuve)
- Mechanism: direct trauma, indirect varus/valgus stress to the knee
- Exam: localized tenderness

Associated Injury
- Lateral condylar fracture
- Common peroneal nerve injury (see Chapter 14)
- Anterior tibial artery injury
- Ligamentous injuries

Radiographic Evaluation
- AP and lateral views
- Consider ankle AP, lateral, and mortise views

Management
- Immobilization in knee immobilizer (for comfort)
- Weight bearing as tolerated with crutches

Disposition
- Isolated fracture: ED discharge and follow-up with orthopedic specialist

KNEE DISLOCATION

General
- Dissociation of articular surfaces of the femur and tibia
  — High risk of concurrent popliteal artery injury
- Classification: anterior (most common), posterior, lateral, medial, rotary (least common)
- Mechanism: high-energy (MVC, fall from height), hyperextension, axial/posterior load to flexed knee (dashboard injury)
- Exam: often spontaneously reduce, can have gross instability, effusion, diminished distal pulses, neurologic injury (foot drop/paresthesia)

Associated Injuries
- Popliteal artery/peroneal nerve (see Chapter 14)
- Tibia/fibula fracture
- Hip dislocation/fractures

Radiographic Evaluation
- AP and lateral views
- CTA to assess for vascular injury

Management

- Immediate reduction by applying longitudinal traction, then anteriorly lifting tibia (if posterior dislocation) or distal femur (if anterior dislocation)
  - Posterolateral dislocations may be irreducible because of entrapment of the joint capsule within the joint
- Immobilization in posterior long-leg splint then vascular assessment (ABI, angiography), non-weight bearing

Disposition

- Discuss with orthopedic specialist while patient is in the ED
  - Almost always requires observation/serial exams or surgical management

LIGAMENT INJURY

Collateral Ligament Injury

General

- Sprain, incomplete tear, or complete rupture of the medial collateral ligament or lateral collateral ligament
- Mechanism
  - MCL: valgus and external rotation stress to flexed knee
  - LCL: varus stress +/- internal rotation
- Exam
  - MCL: joint laxity with valgus stress test
  - LCL: joint laxity with varus stress test

Associated Injuries

- Other ligaments (ACL, PCL), lateral meniscal tears, posterolateral corner injury
- Common or superficial peroneal (fibular) nerve injuries with LCL injuries

Radiographic Evaluation

- AP and lateral views to evaluate for bony injury
  - Arcuate sign: small avulsion from the apex of the fibular head suggestive of LCL injury and likely concurrent PCL injury

Management

- Immobilization in knee immobilizer if significant laxity

Disposition

- ED discharge and follow-up with orthopedic specialist

Cruciate Ligament Injury

General

- Sprain, incomplete tear, or complete rupture of the anterior cruciate ligament (ACL) or posterior cruciate ligament (PCL)
- Mechanism
  - ACL: valgus and external rotation stress to flexed knee, hyperextension stress
  - PCL: posteriorly stress to flexed knee
- Exam
  - ACL: positive anterior drawer and Lachman tests
  - PCL: positive posterior drawer and sag sign

Associated Injuries

- Other ligamentous injuries
- Segond fracture (avulsion fracture of the proximal/lateral tibia) with ACL injury

Radiographic Evaluation

- AP and lateral views to evaluate for bony injury

Management

- Immobilization in knee immobilizer if significant laxity

Disposition

- ED discharge and follow-up with orthopedic specialist

Meniscus Injury

General

- Injury to the medial/lateral meniscus: can be partial tear or complete rupture
- Rare in children < 10 years old
- Mechanism: rotation of flexed knee on a planted foot
- Exam: positive McMurray's, Apley compression, and/or Thessaly tests

Associated Injuries

- Tibial plateau fracture
- ACL/MCL injury

Radiographic Evaluation

- AP and lateral views to evaluate for bony injury

Management

- Immobilization in knee immobilizer if significant laxity

Disposition

- ED discharge and follow-up with orthopedic specialist

OSGOOD-SCHLATTER DISEASE/TIBIAL TUBERCLE APOPHYSITIS (Ⓟ PEDIATRIC)

General

- Overuse injury to the anterior proximal tibial growth plate caused by repeated tensile forces of the quadriceps to the patella tendon insertion on the tibial tuberosity
- Common in young athletes, worse with kneeling or squatting
- Exam: tenderness and swelling over tibial tubercle, pain worse with knee extension against active resistance, effusion uncommon

Associated Injuries

- No commonly associated injuries

Radiographic Evaluation

- Clinical diagnosis, but AP and lateral views may show irregularities of the proximal tibial tuberosity and/or ossicle/calcification in the patellar tendon

Management

- Rest/activity modification

Disposition

- ED discharge and follow-up with pediatrician or pediatric orthopedic specialist

PATELLAR DISLOCATION

General

- Dislocation of patella from patellofemoral groove, most commonly lateral
- Mechanism: forceful contraction of quadriceps with flexed and rotated knee or direct trauma to flexed knee
- Exam: pain worse with knee movement, deformity

Associated Injuries
- Intra-articular loose body or osteochondral fracture of patella
- Fracture of lateral femoral condyle
- Ligamentous injury

Radiographic Evaluation
- AP and lateral views

Management
- Reduction: flex hip, then extend knee while gently pushing the patella back to anatomic position
  — Non-lateral dislocations often require surgical management
- Immobilization in knee immobilizer

Disposition
- Non-lateral dislocations: discuss with orthopedic specialist while patient is in the ED
- All other cases: ED discharge and follow-up with orthopedic specialist

PATELLAR FRACTURE

General
- Considered an intra-articular fracture
- Mechanism: direct trauma to the anterior knee
- Exam: hemarthrosis, palpable deformity, inability to straighten leg
- Bipartite/tripartite patella: congenital anomaly because of patellar bone consisting of two or three separate bones with smooth edges, often misidentified as a fracture

Associated Injuries
- Soft tissue injury
- Quadriceps and/or patellar tendon injury

Radiographic Evaluation
- AP and lateral views
  — Consider sunrise view to differentiate bipartite patella from fracture

Management
- Immobilization in knee immobilizer or posterior long-leg splint
- Weight bearing as tolerated

Disposition
- ED discharge and follow-up with orthopedic specialist

QUADRICEPS AND PATELLAR TENDON RUPTURE

General
- Partial rupture or complete disruption of the quadriceps or patellar tendon
- Mechanism: sudden knee flexion with contracted quadriceps (stepping off a curb)
- Exam: displacement of the patella (inferior if quadriceps tendon injury, superior if patella tendon injury), ability to extend knee decreased or absent

Associated Injuries
- Patella or tibial avulsion fractures
- Ⓟ Patella sleeve fracture: avulsion fracture of the distal patellar pole

Radiographic Evaluation
- AP and lateral views

Management
- Immobilization in knee immobilizer, non-weight bearing

Disposition
- Discuss with orthopedic specialist while patient is in the ED
  - Complete ruptures almost always require surgical management

SINDING-LARSEN-JOHANSSON DISEASE/PATELLAR APOPHYSITIS (Ⓟ PEDIATRIC)

General
- Overuse injury to the inferior pole of the patella caused by repeated stress from the quadriceps on the attachment of the patella tendon on the patella
- Common in young athletes, worse with kneeling or running
- Commonly misidentified as Osgood-Schlatter Disease or patellar tendinitis ("jumper's" knee)
- Exam: pain over the inferior patellar worse with knee extension against active resistance

Associated Injuries
- No commonly associated injuries

Radiographic Evaluation
- Clinical diagnosis, but AP and lateral views may show spurs or blurring of the inferior pole of the patella

Management
- Conservative management

Disposition
- ED discharge and follow-up with pediatrician or pediatric orthopedic specialist

TIBIA EPIPHYSEAL FRACTURE, PROXIMAL (Ⓟ PEDIATRIC)

General
- Typically SH II fracture
- Mechanism: high-energy valgus/varus, and/or hyperextension force to the knee
- Exam: localized tenderness, deformity

Associated Injuries
- Tibial tubercle fracture
- Peroneal artery and/or nerve injury (see Chapter 14)

Radiographic Evaluation
- AP, lateral, and oblique views
  — Consider comparison views

Management
- Immobilization in posterior long-leg splint, non-weight bearing

Disposition
- Discuss with pediatric orthopedic specialist while patient is in the ED
  — Most will require surgical management

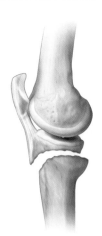

TIBIA METAPHYSEAL/SUBCONDYLAR FRACTURE, PROXIMAL (Ⓟ PEDIATRIC)

General
- Fracture involving the proximal metaphysis of tibia
  — Usually transverse or oblique, can be intra-articular or extra-articular
- Most common age 3–6, but can be seen in adolescents with high-energy mechanisms
- Mechanism: varus/valgus or rotational stress with longitudinal compression
- Exam: localized tenderness, joint effusion if intra-articular

Associated Injuries
- Tibial condylar and plateau fractures

Radiographic Evaluation
- AP and lateral views

Management
- Reduction and immobilization in posterior long-leg splint, non-weight bearing

Disposition
- Discuss with pediatric orthopedic specialist while patient is in the ED
  — Most will require surgical management

TIBIAL PLATEAU FRACTURE

General
- Can be due to high- or low-energy force
- Mechanism: valgus/varus force combined with axial loading
- Exam: pain worse with valgus/varus testing
- Classified as Schatzker Type I–VI

Associated Injuries
- Popliteal artery injury
- Ligamentous injuries and meniscal tears (lateral > medial)
- Compartment syndrome

Radiographic Evaluation
- AP and lateral views

— Oblique and tibial plateau views can help determine level of bone depression
— Increased subchondral bone density suggests tibial plateau fracture
- Consider CT for occult fractures, especially if there is an unexplained knee effusion

Management
- Immobilize in posterior long-leg splint, non-weight bearing
- Indications for surgical management: poly-trauma, comminuted fractures, open fractures, significant soft tissue injury

Disposition
- Discuss with orthopedic specialist while patient is in the ED

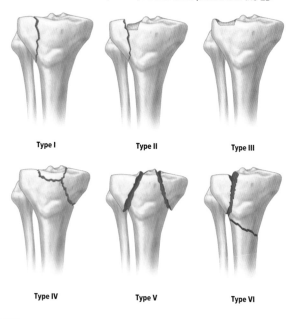

Type I Type II Type III

Type IV Type V Type VI

TIBIAL SHAFT FRACTURE

General
- Most commonly fractured long bone
- Mechanism: typically direct trauma
- Exam: localized tenderness, deformity, inability to bear weight

Associated Injuries
- Peroneal and/or tibial nerve injury (see Chapter 14)
- Vascular injury: rare, so diminished pulses may be sign of compartment syndrome
- Compartment syndrome (see Chapter 14)
  - Most common fracture causing compartment syndrome
  - Consider compartment syndrome in tibial shaft fracture presenting with worsening pain 24–48 hours after casting

Radiographic Evaluation
- AP and lateral views

Management
- Reduction (prior to imaging if neurovascular injury) and immobilization in posterior long-leg splint, non-weight bearing

Disposition
- Discuss with orthopedic specialist while patient is in the ED
  - Almost always requires serial compartment checks +/- surgical management

TIBIAL SPINE/EMINENCE FRACTURE (Ⓟ PEDIATRIC)

General
- Bony avulsion of the ACL from its insertion on the intercondylar eminence
  - Typically occurs in adolescents between ages of 8–14
- Mechanism: valgus and external rotation stress to flexed knee, hyperextension stress
- Exam: pain worse with knee extension, positive anterior drawer test
- Classified as Meyers and McKeever Type I–IV

Associated Injuries
- Ligament and/or meniscus injuries

Radiographic Evaluation

- AP, lateral, and tunnel views
- Consider CT to better visualize fracture and/or MRI to evaluate for ligamentous injury

Management

- Immobilization in posterior long-leg splint with knee in almost full extension, non-weight bearing

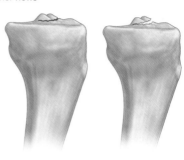

Type I   Type II

Disposition

- Discuss with pediatric orthopedic specialist while patient is in the ED
  - Displaced or completely avulsed fractures almost always require surgical management

TIBIAL TUBEROSITY/TUBERCLE FRACTURE
(Ⓟ PEDIATRIC)

General
- Mechanism: avulsion fracture to due contracted quadriceps opposing sudden knee flexion
- Exam: pain worse with active knee extension
- Classified as Ogden Types I–V

Associated Injuries
- Patellar retinaculum/ligament injury
- Compartment syndrome
- Recurrent anterior tibial artery injury

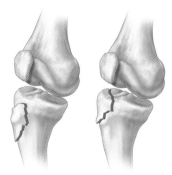

Tibial Tuberosity Fractures

Radiographic Evaluation
- AP and lateral views
  — Consider comparison views

Management
- Immobilization in posterior long-leg splint, non-weight bearing

Disposition
- Discuss with orthopedic specialist while patient is in the ED
  — Most will require surgical management

CHAPTER 11

Ankle

FRACTURES BY LOCATION

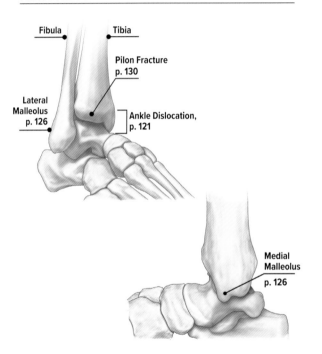

Fibula

Tibia

Pilon Fracture
p. 130

Lateral
Malleolus
p. 126

Ankle Dislocation,
p. 121

Medial
Malleolus
p. 126

OTTAWA ANKLE RULE

- < 15% of ankle injuries have a clinically significant fracture
- Ottawa Ankle Rule can be used to exclude fractures of the ankle and midfoot and reduce X-ray utilization
- Sensitivity is 100% for the Ottawa Ankle Rule with moderate specificity
- Can be used in children > age 6
- **Exclusions:** pregnant women, intoxicated patients, head injuries

Ankle X-ray required if:
- Any pain along malleolar regions AND any of the following:
  — Bony tenderness along distal 6 cm of posterior edge of tibia
  — Bony tenderness at tip of medial malleolus
  — Bony tenderness along distal 6 cm of posterior edge of fibula
  — Bony tenderness at tip of lateral malleolus
  — Inability to bear weight immediately or after 4 steps during evaluation

Foot X-ray required if:
- Any pain in the midfoot region AND any of the following:
  — Bony tenderness at the base of 5th metatarsal
  — Bony tenderness at the navicular
  — Inability to bear weight immediately or after 4 steps during evaluation

ACHILLES TENDON RUPTURE

General
- High misdiagnosis rate because ~33% of patients do not have pain
- Mechanism: sudden forced plantar flexion or excessive dorsiflexion of plantar flexed foot
- Exam: positive Thompson test, plantar flexion weakness

Radiographic Evaluation
- X-rays if concern for bony pathology
- Ultrasound may distinguish between partial and total rupture
- MRI is test of choice if ultrasound is not available

Management
- Assume tendon rupture if suspected but unable to confirm with MRI or ultrasound
- Immobilization in posterior long or short-leg splint or brace with foot in plantar flexion (resting equinus), non-weight bearing

Disposition
- ED discharge and follow-up with orthopedic specialist

ANKLE DISLOCATION

General
- Dissociation of the articular surface of talus from tibia and fibula
- Usually accompanied by fracture(s)
- Isolated dislocation without fracture requires high-energy mechanism
- 4 main categories of dislocations:
  — Anterior
  — Lateral
  — Posterior
  — Superior
- Reduction should be performed prior to imaging if signs of neurovascular injury

Anterior Ankle Dislocation

General
- Exam: foot dorsiflexed and displaced anteriorly

Associated Injuries
- Fracture of the anterior portion of the distal tibia
- Mechanical obstruction of dorsalis pedis artery

Radiographic Evaluation
- AP, lateral, and mortise views

Management
- Reduction and immobilization in posterior short-leg with stirrup splint, non-weight bearing

Anterior Ankle Reduction Technique

Steps	First Person	Second Person
1	Flex the hip and knee to 90°	Provide countertraction at the knee
2	Dorsiflex the foot slightly to disengage the talus then apply axial traction	Apply countertraction
3	Apply anterior force to distal tibia while pushing foot posteriorly to bring back into normal position	Apply countertraction

Disposition
- Discuss with orthopedic specialist while patient is in the ED
  — Almost always requires surgical management

Lateral Ankle Dislocation

General
- Exam: foot displaced laterally

Associated Injuries
- Malleolar (medial and/or lateral) and distal fibula fractures
- Deltoid ligament injury

Radiographic Evaluation
- AP, lateral, and mortise views

Management
- Reduction and immobilization in posterior short-leg with stirrup splint, non-weight bearing

Lateral Ankle Reduction Technique

Steps	First Person	Second Person
1	Flex the hip and knee to 90°	Provide countertraction at the knee
2	Provide axial traction with one hand on the heel and the other on the dorsum of the foot	Apply countertraction
3	Manipulate medially to bring the ankle back into normal position	Apply countertraction
4	Foot and leg can be suspended to allow gravity and ankle position to aid in reduction	Apply countertraction

Disposition
- Discuss with orthopedic specialist while patient is in the ED
  — Almost always requires surgical management

Posterior Ankle Dislocation

General
- Exam: foot plantarflexed and displaced posteriorly
Associated Injuries
- Lateral malleolus fracture
- Disruption of tibiofibular syndesmosis
Radiographic Evaluation
- AP, lateral, and mortise views
Management
- Reduction and immobilization in posterior short-leg with stirrup splint, non-weight bearing

Posterior Ankle Reduction Technique

Steps	First Person	Second Person
1	Flex the hip and knee to 90°	Provide countertraction at the knee
2	Grasp heel with one hand, and dorsum of foot with the other	Apply countertraction
3	Provide axial traction while plantarflexing the foot	Apply countertraction
4	Dorsiflex the foot and pull the heel forward while pushing the tibia posteriorly	Apply countertraction

Disposition
- Discuss with orthopedic specialist while patient is in the ED
  — Almost always requires surgical management

Superior Ankle Dislocation

General
- Uncommon, complete disruption of joint
- Exam: shortened limb with obvious deformity

Associated Injuries
- Articular damage
- Thoracolumbar and/or calcaneal fractures

Radiographic Evaluation
- AP, lateral, and mortise views

Management
- Immobilization in posterior short-leg with stirrup splint

Disposition
- Discuss with orthopedic specialist while patient is in the ED
  — Always requires surgical management

ANKLE FRACTURE (ⓟ PEDIATRIC)

General
- Children more likely to sustain fracture than sprain
- Fracture patterns vary with age
  - Tillaux fracture: Salter-Harris III of the of the distal tibial epiphysis seen in adolescents (12–15 years old)
- Exam: localized tenderness, ecchymosis, deformity

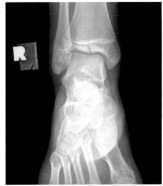

Pediatric Tillaux Fracture

Associated Injuries
- Growth plate injuries
- Tibia and/or fibula fractures

Radiographic Evaluation
- AP, lateral, and mortise views
  - Consider comparison views if concern for Salter-Harris V
- Consider CT for occult fractures

Management
- Reduction and immobilization in posterior short-leg with stirrup splint for confirmed or suspected fractures, non-weight bearing

Disposition
- Discuss with pediatric orthopedic specialist while patient is in the ED
  - Salter-Harris III, IV, and V generally require surgical management

ANKLE/MALLEOLUS FRACTURE

General

- Fractures involving any combination of the following:
  - Medial malleolus: medial aspect of the distal tibia
  - Lateral malleolus: distal fibula
  - Posterior malleolus: posterior aspect of the distal tibia
- Ankle fractures and ligamentous injuries frequently occur together
- Mechanism: forced external rotation/AD-duction of supinated foot (most common) or forced eversion/AB-duction of pronated foot
- Exam: localized tenderness, deformity
- Categorized as:
  - Isolated lateral
  - Isolated medial
  - Bimalleolar (medial + lateral)
  - Trimalleolar (medial + lateral + posterior)
- Widened mortise on plain films suggests deltoid ligament injury and a presumed medial malleolar fracture
- Consider CT for occult fractures and/or MRI for ligamentous injuries

Malleolar Reduction Technique

Steps	First Person	Second Person
1	Flex the hip and knee to 90°	Provide countertraction at the knee
2	Grasp heel with one hand, and forefoot with the other	Apply countertraction
3	Apply axial traction/countertraction and return the talus into a reduced position	Apply countertraction

Lateral Malleolus Fracture

General
- Isolated fractures are stable

Associated Injuries
- Deltoid ligament or tibiofibular syndesmosis injury (either makes ankle unstable)

Radiographic Evaluation
- AP, lateral, and mortise views

Management
- Immobilization in posterior short-leg with stirrup splint, non-weight bearing

Disposition
- Discuss with orthopedic specialist while patient is in the ED

Medial Malleolus Fracture

General
- Isolated fractures usually stable

Associated Injuries
- Deltoid and tibiofibular syndesmotic ligament injury
- Fibular neck fractures (Maisonneuve fracture)
- Lateral or posterior malleolus injury
- Injury to the tibial nerve (see Chapter 14), posterior tibial artery

Radiographic Evaluation
- AP, lateral, and mortise views

Management
- Reduction and immobilization in posterior short-leg with stirrup splint, non-weight bearing

Disposition
- Discuss with orthopedic specialist while patient is in the ED

Bimalleolar Fracture

General
- Unstable fracture of both lateral and medial malleoli
  - Bimalleolar equivalent: lateral malleolar fracture with widened mortise concerning for deltoid ligament injury

Associated Injuries
- Deltoid and tibiofibular syndesmotic ligament injury
- Proximal fibula fracture (Maisonneuve fracture)
- Injury to the tibial nerve (see Chapter 14), posterior tibial artery

Radiographic Evaluation
- AP, lateral, and mortise views

Management
- Reduction and immobilization in posterior short-leg with stirrup splint, non-weight bearing

Disposition
- Discuss with orthopedic specialist while patient is in the ED
  - Almost always requires surgical management

Trimalleolar Fracture

General
- Unstable fracture of lateral (purple arrow), medial (green arrow), and posterior malleoli (yellow arrow)
  - Trimalleolar equivalent: lateral and posterior malleolar fractures with widened mortise concerning for deltoid ligament injury

Associated Injuries
- Deltoid ligament rupture
- Fibular neck fractures
- Injury to the tibial nerve (see Chapter 14), posterior tibial artery, peroneal artery

Radiographic Evaluation
- AP, lateral, and mortise views

Management
- Reduction and immobilization in posterior short-leg with stirrup splint, non-weight bearing

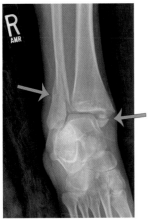
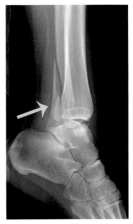

Mortise View   **Lateral View**

Trimalleolar Fracture

Disposition

- Discuss with orthopedic specialist while patient is in the ED
  — Almost always requires surgical management

MAISONNEUVE FRACTURE

General

- Unstable ankle injury that includes a proximal fibula fracture (blue arrow), distal tibiofibular syndesmosis injury, and deltoid ligament rupture (orange arrow) or medial malleolus fracture if deltoid ligament remains intact
- Mechanism: internal rotation of the leg and external rotation of the talus with a planted foot
- Exam: tenderness over proximal fibula and medial ankle

Associated Injuries

- Medial malleolus avulsion fracture
- Ankle ligamentous injuries

Radiographic Evaluation
- AP, lateral, and mortise views
  — Widened mortise suggests deltoid ligament injury (pink arrow)
- Full length tibia or proximal tibia views

Management
- Reduction if displaced (same technique as for malleolar fractures, see p. 126) and immobilization in posterior long-leg with stirrup splint, non-weight bearing

Disposition
- Discuss with orthopedic specialist while patient is in the ED
  — Almost always requires surgical management

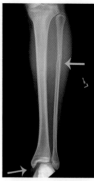

Maisonneuve Fracture

PILON/TIBIAL PLAFOND FRACTURE

General
- Intra-articular fracture(s) of the distal tibia caused when tibia is driven down into the talus bone
- Mechanism: from axial loading (such as jumping from height and landing on the feet)
  — Fracture pattern depends on foot position on impact
- Exam: pain worse with ankle movement, deformity

Associated Injuries
- High risk for compartment syndrome
- Thoracolumbar and/or calcaneal fractures
- Fibula fractures

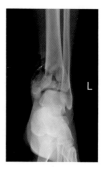

Radiographic Evaluation
- AP, lateral, and mortise views
- Consider CT to better evaluate injury pattern

Management
- Immobilization in posterior short-leg with stirrup splint, non-weight bearing

Disposition
- Discuss with orthopedic specialist while patient is in the ED
  — Most will require surgical management

TODDLER'S FRACTURE (Ⓟ PEDIATRIC)

General
- Isolated non-displaced spiral fracture of the distal half of the tibial shaft in children < 3 years old
- Mechanism: low-energy force with rotational component
  — There may not be a specific history of trauma
- Exam: pain with ankle dorsiflexion or torsional force

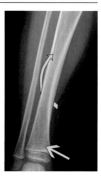

Associated Injuries
- Fibula fracture
- Compartment syndrome is rare

Radiographic Evaluation
- Leg AP and lateral views
  — Fracture may not be present on initial X-rays
- Consider ipsilateral knee and ankle views

Management
- Immobilization in posterior long-leg splint, non-weight bearing

Disposition:
- Discuss with pediatric orthopedic specialist while patient is in the ED

TRIPLANE FRACTURE (🅟 PEDIATRIC)

General
- Can be thought of as a Salter-Harris IV fracture of the distal tibia with a coronal fracture line through the metaphysis, axial fracture through the physis, and sagittal fracture through the epiphysis
  — Similar to Tillaux fracture, but coronal fracture extends through the metaphysis
  — Occurs as the epiphysial plate is closing, usually 10–17 years of age
- Mechanism: ankle inversion/supination with external rotation
- Exam: pain worse with ankle movement, deformity
- May be in 2-, 3-, or 4-part fractures
- 2-part fracture (most common)
  — SH IV fracture pattern seen on lateral view
  — Occurs when medial portion of the distal tibial epiphysis is closed
- 3-part fracture
  — Combination of SH II (seen on lateral view) and SH III (seen on AP view)
  — Occurs when only the middle portion of the distal tibial epiphysis is closed

Associated Injuries
- Spiral fractures of the fibula
- Ipsilateral tibial shaft fracture

Radiographic Evaluation
- AP, lateral, and mortise views
  — Epiphysis fracture often lateral (same as Tillaux fracture), best seen on AP view
  — Metaphyseal fracture often posterior, best seen on lateral view
- CT usually required to better evaluate the fracture pattern

Management

- Reduction (if significant displacement) and immobilization in posterior long-leg with stirrup splint, non-weight bearing

Triplane Reduction Technique

Steps	First Person	Second Person
1	Flex the hip and knee to 90°	Provide stabilization and countertraction at the knee
2	Push lateral fracture segments onto tibia then apply longitudinal traction	
3	Maintain traction and apply pressure to base of tibia	
4	Position foot in external rotation for medial fractures and internal rotation for lateral fractures	

Disposition

- Discuss with pediatric orthopedic specialist while patient is in the ED

CHAPTER **12**

Foot

FRACTURES BY LOCATION

Distal, Middle, Proximal Phalanx
- Fracture, p. 146
- Dislocation, p. 148

Metatarsals
- Fracture, p. 141

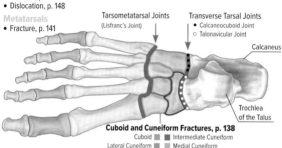

Tarsometatarsal Joints (Lisfranc's Joint)

Transverse Tarsal Joints
- • Calcaneocuboid Joint
- ○ Talonavicular Joint

Calcaneus

Trochlea of the Talus

Cuboid and Cuneiform Fractures, p. 138
- Cuboid ■ ■ Intermediate Cuneiform
- Lateral Cuneiform ■ ■ Medial Cuneiform
- ■ Navicular

Talus Fractures, p. 146

Neck of Talus

Head of Talus

Medial Malleolar Surface

Toe Fracture, p. 146

Navicular Fracture, p. 137

Calcaneal Body Fracture, p. 136

Sesamoid Fracture, p. 147

CALCANEAL BODY FRACTURES/EXTRA-ARTICULAR CALCANEAL FRACTURE

General
- Fracture of the calcaneus ("heel bone") that forms the foundation of the rear part of the foot
- Mechanism: typically fall/jump from significant height
- Exam: may show heel hematoma (Mondor sign)

Associated Injuries
- Extension into the calcaneocuboid joint
- Thoracolumbar injuries (associated with traumatic axial load)
- Contralateral calcaneus fracture
- Compartment syndrome

Radiographic Evaluation
- AP, lateral, and oblique views of the foot
- Assess Bohler's angle
  - Specific but not sensitive for calcaneal fracture
  - Angle between 2 lines on lateral ankle X-ray
    - Line 1 connects the superior margin of the posterior process of the calcaneus to the superior point of the posterior facet
    - Line 2 connects the superior tip of the posterior facet to the superior tip of the anterior facet
    - Normal is 20–40° (< 20° is specific for calcaneus fracture)

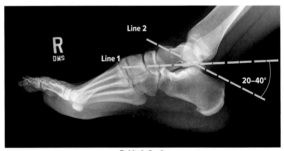

Bohler's Angle

- — Assess for tuberosity elevation
- — Consider Broden, Harris, and AP ankle views
- CT is gold standard and should be done if concern for intra-articular extension

Management
- Reduction and immobilization in posterior short-leg with stirrup splint with bulky heel padding, non-weight bearing
  - — If there is tuberosity elevation, splint in plantar flexion as tolerated

Disposition
- Discuss with orthopedic specialist while patient is in the ED
  - — Most will require surgical management or serial compartment checks

MIDFOOT FRACTURE

General
- Fractures involving the navicular, cuboid, or 3 cuneiform bones
- Typically involve multiple fractures or fracture-dislocations

Navicular Fracture

General
- Most common fractured bone in the midfoot
- Mechanism: usually due to trauma or rotational forces, also can be stress fracture
- Exam: pain worse with foot eversion or pushing off
- Subtypes include
  - — Dorsal avulsion fractures (most common)
    - Os tibiale externa can be mistaken for an avulsion fracture
  - — Tuberosity fractures
  - — Body fractures
  - — Compression fractures

Associated Injuries
- Injury to adjacent structures is common with all navicular fractures
- Dorsal avulsion fractures associated with lateral malleolar ligament injuries

- Tuberosity fractures associated with cuboid fractures and susceptible to nonunion
- Body fractures are susceptible to avascular necrosis and traumatic arthritis

Radiographic Evaluation
- AP, lateral, and oblique views
  — Oblique view best for visualizing tuberosity fractures
- Consider CT for determining displacement in navicular body fractures

Management
- Reduction and immobilization in posterior short-leg with stirrup splint, non-weight bearing

Disposition
- Discuss with orthopedic specialist while patient is in the ED

Cuboid and Cuneiform Fractures

General
- Fracture of the cuboid and/or cuneiform bones, usually occur together
- Isolated fractures are uncommon
- Mechanism: direct trauma, axial load, or forced inversion
- Exam: pain over dorsolateral (cuboid) or dorsal/dorsomedial (cuneiforms) midfoot worse with weight bearing

Associated Injuries
- Fractures of 4th and 5th metatarsal bases
- Cuboid fractures associated with calcaneus fractures
- Lisfranc injuries

Radiographic Evaluation
- AP, lateral, and oblique views
  — Cuboid best visualized on medial oblique view
  — Cuneiforms best visualized on lateral and lateral oblique views
- Consider CT to better visualize fracture pattern

Management
- Immobilization in posterior short-leg with stirrup splint, non-weight bearing

Disposition

- Discuss with orthopedic specialist while patient is in the ED
  — Most will require surgical management, especially if concurrent injuries

Lisfranc Injury

General

- Disruption of the tarsometatarsal (Lisfranc) joint complex
  — Includes articulation of the midfoot (cuboid and cuneiforms) and metatarsals
- Can by purely ligamentous injuries or fracture-dislocations
  — Ligaments include tarsometatarsal, intermetatarsal, and Lisfranc
- Mechanism: typically rotational and axial load on plantarflexed foot
- Exam: plantar ecchymosis, positive pronation-AB-duction test, positive tarsometatarsal squeeze test, positive piano key sign

Associated Injuries

- Avulsion fractures of contiguous tarsals or metatarsals
- Fracture at base of 2nd metatarsal

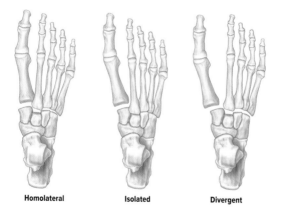

Homolateral   Isolated   Divergent

- Adjacent tarsal bone fractures
- Compartment syndrome if high-energy mechanism

Radiographic Evaluation
- AP, lateral, and oblique views
  - AP view to evaluate for:
    - Alignment of the medial borders of the second metatarsal and middle cuneiform
    - Alignment of the first metatarsal with the borders of the medial cuneiform
    - Bases of the first and second metatarsals should be less than 3 mm apart
    - "Fleck sign": avulsed fragment between bases of 1st and 2nd metatarsals indicating spontaneously reduced dislocation
  - Oblique view to evaluate for:
    - Alignment of the medial borders of the fourth metatarsal and cuboid
    - Alignment of the lateral borders of the third metatarsal and lateral cuneiform
  - Lateral view to evaluate for:
    - Metatarsal dislocation (a metatarsal should never be more dorsal than its associated tarsal)
  - A fracture of the base of the 2nd metatarsal is a Lisfranc fracture-dislocation until proven otherwise
  - Any disruption of the alignment of the medial middle cuneiform and the 2nd metatarsal suggests a spontaneously reduced fracture-dislocation
- Weight bearing views specific but not sensitive
- Consider CT for occult fractures

Management
- Immobilization in posterior short-leg with stirrup splint, non-weight bearing

Disposition
- Discuss with orthopedic specialist while patient is in the ED
  - Fracture-dislocations almost always require surgical management

METATARSAL FRACTURE

First Metatarsal Fracture

General
- Mechanism: typically a direct crush injury
- Exam: pain worse with axial compression or weight bearing

Associated Injuries
- Other metatarsal and/or tarsal fractures
- Foot compartment syndrome
- Medial plantar artery and nerve injury (uncommon) (see Chapter 14)

Radiographic Evaluation
- AP, lateral, and oblique views

Management
- Immobilization in posterior short-leg splint, non-weight bearing

Disposition
- Discuss with orthopedic specialist while patient is in the ED
  - Displaced neck and highly comminuted fractures almost always require surgical management

2nd, 3rd, 4th, and middle/distal 5th Metatarsal Fracture

General
- Mechanism: typically a direct crush injury
- Exam: pain worse with axial compression or weight bearing

Associated Injuries
- Foot compartment syndrome
- Phalanx fractures
- Lisfranc injury, especially if metatarsal base fracture(s) are present
- Neurovascular injury uncommon, assess medial and lateral plantar artery and nerve (see Chapter 14)

Radiographic Evaluation
- AP, lateral, and oblique views

Management
- Isolated non-displaced fractures: hard-sole shoe, weight bearing as tolerated
- Displaced > 3 mm or angulated > 10° fractures
  - Reduction using traction (finger traps)/countertraction (weights hung on distal tibia) and immobilization in posterior short-leg splint, non-weight bearing

Disposition
- Discuss with orthopedic specialist while patient is in the ED
  - Multiple fractures usually require surgical management

Proximal 5th Metatarsal Tuberosity Avulsion Fracture (Pseudo-Jones Fracture, Styloid Fracture of the 5th Metatarsal)

General
- Fracture of the base of the 5th metatarsal proximal to its articulation with the 4th metatarsal
  - Often extra-articular but can involve the cuboid-metatarsal joint
  - Most common fracture of the proximal 5th metatarsal
- Normal variant accessory ossicles (os peroneum and os vesalianum) can be mistaken for fracture
- Mechanism: forced inversion of plantarflexed ankle and foot
- Exam: pain worse with horizontal compression of the metatarsal heads

Associated Injuries
- Lateral ankle ligamentous complex injury
- Phalanx fractures

Radiographic Evaluation
- AP, lateral, and oblique views

Management
- Immobilization in posterior short-leg splint, non-weight bearing
  - Can also consider immobilization in short-leg splint, hard-soled shoe/cast, or elastic bandages, weight bearing as tolerated

Disposition

- Discuss with orthopedic specialist while patient is in the ED
  - Surgical management is often required for comminuted fractures or fractures with significant intra-articular involvement

Proximal 5th Metatarsal Fracture (Jones Fracture)

General

- Fracture of the 5th metatarsal at the metaphyseal-diaphyseal junction involving the medial facet that articulates with the 4th metatarsal
  - Usually occurs about 1.5–3 cm distal to the 5th metatarsal tuberosity
- Diaphysis stress fractures occur distal to the articulation of the 4th and 5th metatarsals
- Mechanism: lateral force applied to plantarflexed ankle and foot
- Exam: pain worse with horizontal compression of the metatarsal heads

Associated Injuries

- High risk for non-union
- Lateral ankle ligamentous complex injuries
- Phalanx fractures

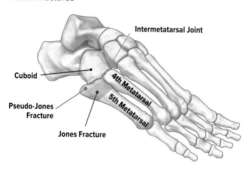

Radiographic Evaluation
- AP, lateral, and oblique views
  - Apophysis runs longitudinal to the shaft, commonly misdiagnosed as a fracture

Management
- Immobilization in posterior short-leg splint, non-weight bearing

Disposition
- Discuss with orthopedic specialist while patient is in the ED
  - Often requires surgical management

Proximal 5th Metatarsal Diaphyseal Stress Fracture

General
- Fracture of the proximal diaphysis of the 5th metatarsal
  - Extends 1.5 cm distally from the metaphyseal-diaphyseal junction
- Mechanism: stress fracture typically seen in athletes
- Exam: pain worse with horizontal compression of the metatarsal heads

Associated Injuries
- Phalanx fractures

Radiographic Evaluation
- AP, lateral, and oblique views

Management
- Immobilization in posterior short-leg splint, non-weight bearing

Disposition
- Discuss with orthopedic specialist while patient is in the ED

SUBTALAR/PERITALAR DISLOCATION

General
- Dislocation of the talus from both the calcaneus and navicular bones
  - Typically medial (most common) or lateral

- Mechanism: forced inversion or eversion of the foot
- Exam: presents with foot locked in supination or pronation

Associated Injuries
- Malleolar, talar, navicular, calcaneal, and/or cuboid fractures
- Talonavicular dislocation

Radiographic Evaluation
- AP, lateral, and oblique views
- Consider post-reduction CT to evaluate for additional injuries (common)

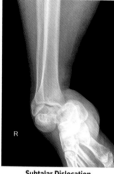

Subtalar Dislocation

Management
- Reduction and immobilization in posterior short-leg with stirrup splint, non-weight bearing
  — Frequently irreducible

Subtalar/Peritalar Reduction Technique

Steps	First Person	Second Person
1	Flex the hip and knee to 90°	Provide countertraction at the knee
2	Apply axial traction to foot and heel	Apply countertraction
3	AB-duct or AD-duct the foot (based on the direction of dislocation) to reestablish anatomical alignment	Apply countertraction

Disposition
- Discuss with orthopedic specialist while patient is in the ED
  — Lateral dislocations often require surgical management

TALUS FRACTURE

General
- Divided into head, neck, and body
  — "Snowboarder's fracture": lateral process fracture
- Often missed on plain films and misdiagnosed as ankle sprains
- Mechanism: high energy injuries leading to axial loading
- Exam: pain worse with ankle movement or weight bearing

Associated Injuries
- Concurrent traumatic injuries (eg, vertebral injuries, ipsilateral lower extremity injuries)
- High risk of avascular necrosis with fracture-dislocations and displaced/comminuted body fractures

Radiographic Evaluation
- AP and lateral views (poor sensitivity)
  — Oblique view may identify subtle subluxation or dislocation
  — Canale view provides optimal view of talar neck
- CT for occult fractures

Management
- Reduction and immobilization in posterior short-leg with stirrup splint molded to support the longitudinal arch, non-weight bearing
  — For posterior process fracture: splint in 15° of plantar flexion

Disposition
- Discuss with orthopedic specialist while patient is in the ED

TOE FRACTURE

General
- Fracture of distal, middle, or proximal phalanx
- Mechanism: axial loading, AB-duction injuries, crush injury
- Exam: pain worse with movement

Associated Injuries
- Nail bed injuries with distal phalanx fractures

Radiographic Evaluation
- AP, lateral, and oblique views

Management

- Reduction (if needed): apply traction and manipulate toe back into anatomical alignment
- Immobilization
  - Non-displaced or minimally displaced fractures: dynamic splinting (buddy taping), hard-soled open shoe, weight bearing as tolerated
  - Comminuted fractures of 1st toe: posterior short-leg splint, non-weight bearing

Disposition

- ED discharge and follow-up with orthopedic specialist for intra-articular or comminuted 1st toe fractures

SESAMOID FRACTURE

General

- Most commonly stress fracture from overuse among athletes
- Mechanism: direct blow or hyper-dorsiflexion of the foot usually at the first MTP
- Exam: tenderness over sesamoid and/or the 1st MTP, pain with dorsiflexion of 1st MTP

Associated Injuries

- Sesamoiditis (inflammation of sesamoid bone)
  - Presents similarly to a fracture, associated with rheumatologic conditions

Radiographic Evaluation

- AP, lateral, and oblique tangential views

Management

- Immobilization in hard-soled open shoe or posterior short-leg splint
- Weight bearing as tolerated

Disposition

- ED discharge and follow-up with primary care provider

TOE DISLOCATION

General

- Dislocation of the metatarsophalangeal joints or interphalangeal joints
- Mechanism: axial load and hyperextension/lateral/medial/dorsal forces
- Exam: localized tenderness, limited range of motion, deformity

Associated Injuries

- Phalangeal fractures

Radiographic Evaluation

- AP, lateral, and oblique views

Management

- Reduction: apply traction and manipulate toe back into anatomical alignment
- Immobilization with dynamic splinting (buddy taping), hard-soled open shoe, weight bearing as tolerated
- Indications for surgical management: irreducible/unstable reductions, post-reduction intra-articular bodies

Disposition

- ED discharge and follow-up with orthopedic specialist

CHAPTER 13

Splinting

Adapted from EMRA Splinting Techniques Guide

Splint Layers
- Inner: stockinette and padding (be generous)
- Middle: plaster or fiberglass
- Outer: compressive dressing/bandaging

Materials
- Stockinette
- Splinting material
  - Plaster: 8–10 layers for upper extremity, 10–12 layers for lower extremity
  - Prefabricated fiberglass
- Padding
- Elastic bandaging
- Bucket/receptacle of water (the warmer the water, the faster the splint sets)
- Trauma shears

Measuring
- Length: measure out the dry splint on the contralateral extremity
- Width: slightly greater than the diameter of the limb

Procedure
1. Apply the stockinette to extend 2" beyond the splinting material; cut holes for finger(s) as needed
2. Apply several layers of padding over the area to be splinted and between digits being splinted; add an extra 2–3 layers over bony prominences

3. Apply lightly moistened splinting material and fold the ends of stockinette over the splinting material
4. Apply the elastic bandaging
5. While still wet, use palms to mold the splint to the desired shape
6. Once hardened, check neurovascular status and motor function

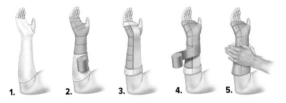

1. **2.** **3.** **4.** **5.**

Complications
- Compartment syndrome
- Ischemia
- Neurologic injury
- Thermal injury
- Pressure sores, skin breakdown
- Infection
- Dermatitis
- Joint stiffness

POSTERIOR LONG-ARM

Indications
- Olecranon fractures
- Humerus fractures
- Radial head and/or neck fractures

Procedure
- Start at posterior proximal arm, down the ulnar forearm, end at MCP joints

Positioning
- Elbow flexed 90°
- Forearm in neutral position with thumb up
- Wrist extended 10–20° (as if holding a can)

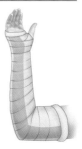

VOLAR

Indications
- Soft tissue injuries of the hand and wrist
- Carpal bone fractures
- 2nd-5th metacarpal head fractures

Procedure
- Start at metacarpal heads and end at distal forearm

Positioning
- Forearm in neutral position with thumb up
- Wrist extended 10–20° (as if holding a can)

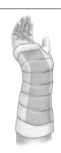

SUGAR TONG

Indications
- Distal radius and/or ulna fractures

Procedure
- Start at dorsal metacarpal heads and end at volar MCP joints

Positioning
- Elbow flexed 90°
- Forearm in neutral position with thumb up
- Wrist extended 10–20° (as if holding a can)

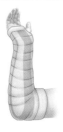

DOUBLE SUGAR TONG

Indications
- Complex and unstable forearm fractures
- Elbow fractures

Procedure
- Forearm sugar-tong splint (place 1st): start at dorsal metacarpal heads and end at volar MCP joints
- Arm sugar-tong splint: start at medial proximal humerus, wrap around elbow, end at lateral proximal humerus

Positioning
- Elbow flexed 90°
- Forearm in neutral position with thumb up
- Wrist extended 10–20° (as if holding a can)

RADIAL GUTTER

Indications
- 2nd and 3rd digit fractures and/or soft tissue injuries
- 2nd and 3rd metacarpal fractures of the neck, shaft, and/or base

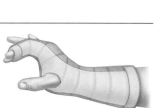

Procedure
- Start at radial side of mid-forearm, end at mid-distal phalanx of 2nd and 3rd digits

Positioning
- Forearm in neutral position
- Wrist extended 10–20° (as if holding a can)
- Thumb AB-ducted
- MCP flexed 50–70° (90° for metacarpal neck fractures)
- Proximal interphalangeal and distal interphalangeal joints flexed 5–10° (as if holding a can)

THUMB SPICA

Indications
- Injuries to scaphoid, lunate, thumb and 1st metacarpal
- Gamekeeper's/skier's thumb
- de Quervain's tenosynovitis

Procedure
- Start at mid-distal phalanx of thumb, end at mid-forearm

Positioning
- Forearm in neutral position
- Wrist extended 10–20° (as if holding a can)
- Thumb AB-ducted (as if holding a wineglass)

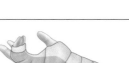

ULNAR GUTTER

Indications
- 5th digit fractures and/ or soft tissue injuries
- 4th and 5th metacarpal fractures of the neck, shaft, and/or base

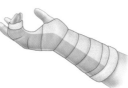

Procedure
- Start at ulnar side of mid-forearm, end at mid-distal phalanx of 4th and 5th digits

Positioning
- Forearm in neutral position
- Wrist extended 10–20° (as if holding a can)
- MCP flexed 50–70° (90° for boxer's fracture)
- Proximal and distal interphalangeal joints flexed 5–10°

FINGER

Indications
- Phalanx fractures and/or dislocations
- PIP or MCP dislocations
- Tendon injuries

Procedure

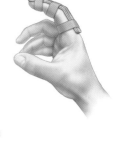

- Typically use prefabricated splint cut to size
- Can be placed on dorsal or volar side, extending from fingertip to mid-hand or distal forearm depending on the joints requiring immobilization

Positioning
- MCP flexed 50°
- Proximal and distal interphalangeal joints flexed 15–20°
- For tendon repairs injuries, splint in flexion or extension as indicated

MALLET FINGER

Indications
- Mallet finger

Placement

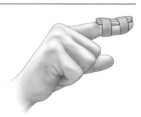

- Splint only the distal interphalangeal joint on dorsal side

Positioning
- Dorsal splinting requires full extension (not hyperextension)

POSTERIOR KNEE

Indications
- Patella fracture and/or dislocation
- Patella or quadriceps tendon injury
- Soft tissue injuries of the knee
- Patients with legs too large for knee immobilizer

Procedure
- Start just distal to gluteal fold, end approximately 6 cm above the malleoli

Positioning
- Knee flexed 15–20°

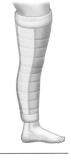

POSTERIOR LEG (SHORT AND LONG)

Indications
- Short-leg with stirrup
  - Calcaneus fractures
  - Talus fractures
  - Ankle fractures, dislocations, and/or sprains
  - Metatarsal fractures
  - Midfoot fractures
  - Achilles tendon injuries
- Long-leg
  - Knee dislocations
  - Tibial plateau fractures
  - Tibia fractures
  - Distal femur fractures

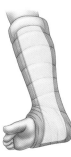

Procedure

- Short-leg: with patient prone, start at plantar surface of the metatarsal heads (base of the toes) and end at the level of the fibular head (just below the knee)
- Stirrup: place after short-leg, start 3–4 cm below the level of fibular head, extend under the plantar surface of foot, end at starting height on contralateral side of leg
- Long-leg: start distal to the gluteal fold and end at base of the toes

Positioning

- Short-leg: ankle in neutral position (90° to leg)
- Achilles injuries: ankle plantarflexed 20–30°
  — Have patient hang leg off table (while sitting up) and ankle will naturally relax to this position
- Long-leg: ankle in neutral position (90° to leg) with knee flexed 15–20°

This splinting primer was adapted from the EMRA Splinting Techniques Guide by R. Ian Ross, MD, with reviewer Anna L. Waterbrook, MD, FACEP, CAQ-SM.

CHAPTER 14

Neurologic Exam

SPINAL INJURY EVALUATION

General
- Injury to the spinal cord, cauda equina, or nerve roots
- Testing should always include sensory and motor
  - Testing light touch is not a formal test of dermatomes
- Test spinal level rather than individual nerve roots
  - Deficits identified in multiple spinal and/or peripheral nerve levels suggests spinal cord, nerve root, and/or plexus (brachial/lumbosacral) injury

Myotomes	
C5	Shoulder abduction
C6	Elbow flexion, wrist extension
C7	Elbow extension, wrist flexion
C8	Finger flexion
T1	Finger abduction/adduction, thumb opposition
L1, L2, L3	Hip flexion
L2, L3	Hip adduction
L3, L4	Knee extension
L4	Ankle dorsiflexion
L5	Hallux dorsiflexion
S1	Ankle eversion, plantar flexion

Dermatomes	
C2	Occiput
C3	Neck
C4	Upper shoulder
C5	Lateral shoulder
C6	Thumb
C7	Middle finger
C8	Little finger
T1	Inner arm
T4-T5	Nipple
T10	Umbilicus
L1	Inguinal fold, scrotum
L2	Lateral thigh
L3	Knee
L4	Inner leg, medial malleolus
L5	Outer leg, dorsum of the foot
S1	Lateral foot and heel
S2, S3	Dorsum of legs and thigh
S4, S5	Perineum

Upper Extremity Peripheral Nerve Localization		
Peripheral Nerve	Sensory	Motor
Axillary	Lateral Shoulder	Shoulder abduction
Long Thoracic	—	Push arm forward against resistance
Median	Volar digits 1–3	Thumb opposition
Musculocutaneous	Lateral forearm	Elbow flexion, Forearm supination
Radial	Dorsal first web space	Wrist and elbow extension
Ulnar	Volar digits 4–5	Thumb Adduction; Finger abduction/adduction
Anterior interosseus	—	Make "OK" sign
Posterior interosseus	—	Wrist extension, finger extension at the MCP joints

Lower Extremity Peripheral Nerve Localization		
Peripheral Nerve	**Sensory**	**Motor**
Sciatic	Common peroneal + tibial nerve distributions (see below)	
Femoral	Anterior thigh	Knee extension
Saphenous	Medial leg	—
Obturator	Medial thigh	Hip adduction
Tibial	Plantar surface	Plantar flexion
Common Peroneal (Fibular)	Superficial + deep peroneal nerve distributions (see below)	
Superficial Peroneal (Fibular)	Dorsum of foot	Foot eversion
Deep Peroneal (fibular)	Dorsum 1st web space	Foot dorsiflexion, Hallux extension
Lateral Plantar	Lateral plantar surface	—
Medial Plantar	Medial plantar surface	—

Motor Strength Grading	
Grade	**Description**
0/5	No muscle movement
1/5	Visible muscle contraction, but no movement at the joint
2/5	Movement at the joint, but not against gravity
3/5	Movement against gravity, but not against added resistance
4/5	Movement against resistance, but less than normal
5/5	Normal strength

Reflexes

- Upper motor neuron lesion: hyperreflexia (except if neurogenic/spinal shock), hypertonicity, spasticity
- Lower motor neuron lesion: areflexia/hyporeflexia, hypotonicity, flaccidity

DTR Grading	
Grade	Description
0	Absent
1+ or +	Hypoactive
2+ or ++	Normal
3+ or +++	Hyperactive without clonus
4+ or ++++	Hyperactive with clonus

DTR Localization	
Spinal Nerve Root and Segment	Reflex Tested
C5	Biceps
C6	Brachioradialis
C7	Triceps
L4	Patellar
S1	Achilles (calcaneal)

Cord Syndromes

Syndrome	Mechanism	Symptoms
Anterior cord	• Hyperflexion injuries • Injury to anterior spinal artery	• Bilateral loss of motor, temperature, and pain below lesion • Proprioception and vibration sense preserved
Central cord	Hyperextension injuries	• Quadriparesis (upper > lower) below lesion • +/- Loss of pain and temperature (upper > lower) below lesion
Brown-Sequard	• Transverse hemisection of spinal cord • Lateral mass fractures	• Ipsilateral spastic paralysis, loss of proprioception and vibration sense below lesion • Contralateral loss of pain and temperature 1–2 levels below lesion

COMPARTMENT SYNDROME

General
- Irreversible muscle injury because of vascular insufficiency caused by localized swelling in muscle groups enclosed by fascial sheaths
- Most common locations are leg and forearm
- Most common cause is fracture
- Coagulopathies increase risk

Clinical Features
- Pain that is persistent, not alleviated with immobilization, and worse with passive stretching
- Diminished sensation to light touch and/or two-point discrimination

Evaluation
- Compartment pressures measured with commercially developed devices
  - Measure within 5 cm of fracture site
- Normal pressures are < 10 mmHg
  - Traditional cutoff for fasciotomy is > 30 mmHg
  - Alternative cutoff: Diastolic blood pressure—compartment pressure < 20–30 mmHg

Treatment
- Remove all splints/dressings and place limb at level of the heart
  - Minimize flexion if elbow or forearm involvement
- Fasciotomy
  - Ischemic damage is irreversible after ~8 hours

Index